LEE,

THANK YOU FOR YOUR
FRIENDSHIP! I AM
SO HAPPY WE ARE
FRIENDS. WELCOME TO
BEING FITFAB!!!

— RICHARD

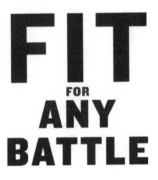

TRAIN YOUR BODY + MIND FOR
LIFE AFTER 40

FIT

FOR
ANY
BATTLE

RICHARD BAGDONAS

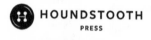

Fit for Any Battle

Train Your Body + Mind for Life After 40

ISBN   978-1-5445-2650-8 *Hardcover*
      978-1-5445-2648-5 *Paperback*
      978-1-5445-2649-2 *Ebook*

CONTENTS

AUTHOR'S NOTE

Thank you for picking up a copy of my book. The Fit for Any Battle (a.k.a "FitFAB") Workout started out as a hypothesis for how to reduce the injuries that had plagued my workouts since I turned forty. I knew I could not maintain my weightlifting regimen much longer, and I needed an alternative. I started using myself as a guinea pig, trying various combinations of techniques, which eventually led me to the FitFAB structure. Then I was diagnosed with stage IV cancer. The moment I was diagnosed, I knew I needed fitness as more than just a hobby. My health was now a matter of life and death.

Driven by passion, and a little bit of fear, I discovered that the workout allowed me to heal my body with little to no pain. Anytime I did get injured, the workout structure allowed me to strengthen the muscles around the injured area so they could help support the healing process. Most importantly, this workout helped me save my sanity. I was living in shock every moment after my cancer diagnosis, fearful of leaving my sons without a father and the love of my life without a husband.

A year and a half after my initial diagnosis, along with getting through the mental stress of a cancer diagnosis, the start of cancer treatment, and kicking cancer's butt—I have never felt stronger.

The success of my journey compelled me to share my story with others who may need a routine that helps them resolve the physical and mental struggles they are facing or will face as they get older. This book is my way of sharing the intimate details of my journey, including how this workout changed the course of my journey and saved my life.

I invite you to use the FitFAB Workout to help with anything you may be going through. And if you know someone who could benefit from an injury-free workout routine, I urge you to share this book with them. Together, we can transform into our strongest selves.

Thank you,
Richard Bagdonas

This book is possible because of
the love and heroic efforts of my beautiful wife,
Tina, and the love of our two sons, Alec and Sky, and
four amazing dogs, Jasper, Tucker, Jellybean, and Muffin.
I love you all very much and still miss you,
Jasper and Tucker.

I am here to write this book because of
Dr. Michael Wang and his amazing team at
the MD Anderson Cancer Center.
Thank you for saving my life!

CHAPTER ONE

MY CANCER JOURNEY

Montezuma's revenge saved my life. That is where my journey writing this book began. My family and I had traveled with some friends to Playa del Carmen, Mexico, to relax and enjoy some time in the sun.

One afternoon, our group stopped at a local restaurant to enjoy some fresh Mexican papaya. What we did not know at the time was that these papayas contained a small protozoon called *Cyclospora cayetanensis*. It is still hard to believe something so small could wreak such havoc. When the discomfort persisted, even after we returned home, I knew I had to call my doctor. Almost immediately, my doctor referred me to a gastroenterologist to determine whether something more than Montezuma's revenge was going on.

The gastroenterologist at Austin Gastroenterology performed a colonoscopy to identify any contributing factors to my intestinal woes. Initially, everything seemed positive. We even laughed together about the small note my wife had written for him on my backside that read, "Be gentle!" He reassured me that everything looked clean. There were no polyps or other signs of colon cancer. He did find some minor inflammation on the walls of my intestines and had taken a few biopsies to double-check it with the lab, but he did not seem worried about it, so I left believing it was all good news.

About three weeks later, the doctor called me to deliver the news. I was still under the impression that everything was fine, but I knew something was off when he started the conversation with, "Sit down." I had just returned home from picking up our youngest son from preschool when he told me, "You have pulled the golden lottery ticket. You have lymphoma!"

I have been in the healthcare industry for over fifteen years. Never once did I associate a cancer diagnosis in the lymphatic system with good news. My previous company was the largest transcription vendor providing services to US Oncology in the state of Texas. I had been around oncologists far too long to think any cancer diagnosis was a good thing.

My personal health journey has been focused on weightlifting since I was fourteen years old. In my late teens, I became a bodybuilder, and that passion for strength and conditioning continued all the way into my forties. I have been a bodybuilder, a runner, and a cyclist, having completed my first Olympic-distance triathlon at thirty years old. At the time of the cancer diagnosis, I had been a vegetarian for several years, given up alcohol, and never smoked a cigarette in my life. I was doing all the right things with diet and exercise.

This was why this diagnosis was good news. Little did I know I had been preparing for cancer my whole life. The strength and conditioning regimen I had been using in my forties, coupled with catching the cancer before it tore through my body, allowed me to survive treatment. My mindset was not just surviving but thriving, and I used the FitFAB Workout regimen to do just that.

Hearing the diagnosis was scary and shocking, but the most terrifying part was breaking the news to my wife, Tina. I knew I had to tell her right away, so I hung up the phone and walked to her office.

I knocked on the door, sat down, and explained to her that her husband of nine years had cancer. The look on her face was what one would expect, a combination of fear and pain. Almost immediately, Tina sprang into action, Googling everything she could on mantle cell lymphoma (MCL).

Do not Google "mantle cell lymphoma" until after you have read this chapter. Everything you read online will be very morbid, but it is simply old data. Things in oncology change so fast that medical journals should be considered history books rather than relevant articles on the latest in medical science.

The data available on Google do not represent what is possible for MCL patients. Today, most patients do not die from MCL. Research and treatments funded by the Cancer Prevention and Research Institute of Texas and the Obama administration's Cancer Moonshot program have made the disease highly treatable. MCL was, at the time of my diagnosis, commonly brought into remission with a series of chemotherapy, radiation, and medications. But this was all information we learned much later.

The day we found out about my diagnosis, Tina and I Googled ourselves into hysteria. We started circulating the news to our close friends and family. Having been in healthcare technology for close to two decades, I had built many friendships with other healthcare folks. The goal was to figure out how we could get me help right away. We decided to wait until after we knew more about the situation before sharing the news with our two boys, Alec and Sky, who were six and three years old, respectively. Thankfully, we did not have to wait long.

My wife's mother, Peggy, had a friend, Jerry, who had MCL and was seen by a doctor at MD Anderson in Houston, Texas. I have always known MD Anderson as "the" place to go for US cancer care. Jerry agreed to talk to me, and after our initial phone call, he provided me with the name and email address for his oncologist at MD Anderson.

I then crafted an email that would ultimately have a role in saving my life. It read as follows.

Dear Dr. Wang,

Good afternoon and please forgive the unannounced email. My name is Richard Bagdonas. It was recommended that I contact you by one of your former patients because I was diagnosed yesterday with early-stage mantle cell lymphoma.

Some demographics on me: forty-five-year-old male who does not drink, smoke, or eat meat. I work out six days a week and feel that I am in good health.

It came as a shock during a colonoscopy that they found cells in my intestine that tested positive for mantle cell lymphoma.

Jerry told me that you specialize in this type of cancer, and I would like to know if you would be willing to meet with me. I live in Austin, Texas, and my in-laws live in Houston, so I can camp out there for a bit if needed. I have an appointment on Monday with Texas Oncology in Austin.

Kindly let me know if you would be willing to meet. My cell phone is ###-###-#### in case you want to call me. Thank you, sir.

I received a response from Dr. Wang the very next morning, and he indicated he would indeed like to see me. Unbeknownst to me, and at the same time that I was writing that email, Tina was on the phone with her business partner. They were trying to figure out how to get me into MD Anderson. By way of her business partner's contacts, I was put in touch with someone in the administration of MD Anderson who asked me to call the next day to get an appointment to see Dr. Wang.

A call into the MD Anderson administration office on the morning of Thursday, September 27, 2018, led me to an 8:00 a.m. appointment in Houston just four days later. Getting into MD Anderson in a timely manner is unheard of, and I am thankful and lucky to be surrounded by a network of wonderful folks in healthcare.

My first instinct was to let the people I work with know I was going to be out of the office the following Monday and explain why. The rush of support and understanding was wonderful to see. My work family had my back as I went into what felt like the black box of cancer care.

ENTERING THE BLACK BOX
OF CANCER CARE

Dr. Wang had a calming effect. As soon as he entered the exam room, he took my arm, smiled, and said, "You don't look sick, so why are you here?" This bit of levity was just what I needed to feel safe. He knew what I was thinking, and this was his way of assuring me that everything would be okay.

I asked him if it would be okay to record our exam session on my phone because I wanted Tina to hear the same words that I did and not relay secondhand information to her. He agreed, and I began recording our conversation.

We discussed the initial results of my colonoscopy, and Dr. Wang agreed to be my doctor. He admitted me as his patient and immediately scheduled a variety of tests. For the next twenty-four hours, I submitted to every test imaginable. While it was not a fun experience, I was grateful that the universe put me in the right place and with the right person.

My friend Nick Adkins had started handing out pink socks with black mustaches on them many years ago at healthcare conferences nationwide. His grassroots Twitter movement called #pinksocks celebrates the good that people are doing in the world. I had been given my first pair in 2015 and had gifted many pairs of them myself. I personalize #pinksocks to showcase the providers who treat patients foremost as someone's son, daughter, mom, or dad. I decided at that very first appointment with Dr. Wang that he would be the recipient of the next pair of pink socks, so I reached into my backpack and presented a pair to him with tears in my eyes. This man wanted to save my life, and the socks were my way of recognizing him for what he was doing for my family.

Dr. Wang treated me as a brother rather than a patient. His eyes showed the determination and grit he had in taking on a cancer that had killed or severely weakened everyone it had come across. When Dr. Wang said we would get through this and I would be back to my normal life, I had to believe him, as I had nothing else to clutch to besides the possibility of not making it. I sat in the treatment room at MD Anderson telling myself, *I will follow this man wherever he needs to take me.* He loved me and wanted the best for me, and that type of bedside manner helped me get through the emotional ordeal.

The twenty-four hours of tests started with a simple blood draw at MD Anderson's massive "needle farm," where countless rows of phlebotomists sit waiting to poke the next patient. My name was called, and I sat watching as sticker after sticker printed on a small label printer.

"How many are we pulling today?" I chuckled.

"Eleven," she said, with a small smile and caring eyes.

It turned out to be the easiest test for the foreseeable future. The bone marrow biopsy was scheduled for the following morning.

I will not go into too much detail about my bone marrow biopsy, but let me just say it was the most painful test I have ever had in my life. Without question, it was essential to my journey, and if you are ever in a similar position, it is an important test to take. But make sure they tell you about your option to be under general anesthesia. Take the general anesthesia, and have someone drive you home.

My first experience was without anesthesia. To stop myself from chickening out, I tried to convince myself that the pain was going to save my life. Nervous, I lay on the table so that the doctor could numb the area. The next thing I knew, a huge needle stabbed into my hip. The doctor started to manually turn the needle to get to the center of my bone, where the marrow is made. The entire process was excruciating and a bit gruesome. It went so badly that the doctor had to perform the procedure a second time. The first sample she pulled was unusable. Apparently, all my years as a milk-drinking weightlifter made my bones incredibly dense. So dense that the needle got stuck! Her second try was much more successful. I was under general anesthesia, and everything went smoothly, as far as I know.

After the second procedure, all we could do was wait for the results. This was a time of reflection. Were there loose ends to my life? I wrote down a password list for Tina and put it in a safe place. I made sure our life insurance was up to date and our friends and family knew of the battle we were in. Getting through this was going to be more than physical; it would include a brutal onslaught of mental challenges.

Thankfully, the workout regimen I used allowed me to process the random thoughts that would press on my mind each day. The night I received my diagnosis, I went to the gym. I sat there crying as I thought about what my two sweet boys would do if I left. Inside this book is a process I used then and still use today to clear out the negative thoughts and allow my mind to be quieted, even if for a brief time, at the gym. I refer to it as the FitFAB mental workout. I can attest to its efficacy.

I spent the time making sure everything was in order just in case I was unable to beat cancer. As a healthy person with a fitness background, I did not anticipate needing any of these things for a long time. Because the alternative was for me to simply sit around and wait for a call from my doctor, it was helpful to have things to do.

It would be two weeks before I went back to Houston for a PET scan and to review the results of the various tests I had taken over the course of twenty-four hours. Those two weeks felt like they took forever. I forced myself to stay positive, despite everything Google had told me, because nobody knew what the outcome would be. I had trusted what my body could accomplish up to this point; there was no reason to doubt its abilities now. I likened my situation to Schrödinger's cat; the cancer was either eating me alive or it was sitting quiet. I chose to believe it was sitting quiet and focused my energy on keeping it that way through positive thinking and meditation whereby I used visualization techniques to envision myself cancer-free.

In addition to all the meditation and reflection, I met with another oncologist in Austin. She was a former client of my previous company and came highly recommended by everyone I asked around town. My goal was to have her work in coordination with Dr. Wang's team and provide any necessary treatments in Austin when I could not make it to Houston. I mentioned her to Dr. Wang, and he agreed that I could take some treatments locally, and given the ongoing COVID-19 pandemic, it made sense to spend a lot more time in the Austin office.

I remain grateful for all the work that the Austin oncologist did for me, especially after our less-than-perfect first meeting. In that initial conversation, she was able to see the results from my bone marrow test—results I was still days away from hearing. She thought that I already knew those results, so she casually mentioned that the Houston lab had found mantle cell lymphoma in my bone marrow. My heart sank to the floor.

During my conversation with Dr. Wang, he took time to explain the different stages of MCL cancer to me. He said stage I meant that the tumor was only in a single lymph node. Stage II meant that there were multiple tumors in my lymph nodes and one other area of my body, such as the groin or neck. Stage III meant that there were multiple tumors in various areas of my body. And finally, stage IV, the worst case, meant that the tumors had moved to another system, like the bone marrow.

The Austin oncologist's casual mention of cancer in my bone marrow was a major blow to my psyche. I had spent so much time over the last two weeks imagining the moment I would hear the news that my cancer was super-early stage I MCL. Now I was certain we were in the worst-case scenario.

After that visit, my wife and I shared one of our worst nights of sleep. We lay together, holding hands and sending squeezes of morse code, quietly telling the other that we loved them.

Tina and I drove out to Houston a couple weeks later for my appointment at MD Anderson. The PET scan was to be done at six o'clock the next morning, and instead of sulking in the hotel, we decided to spend that time celebrating. Tina and I got dressed for what turned out to be the most amazing dinner at Nobu with the most beautiful woman. We had an incredible array of sashimi, including my favorite, sea urchin topped with quail eggs. The delicious food and comfort of my wife by my side helped me get some sleep as we waited for morning to arrive.

THE BIG REVEAL

My biggest fear was that Dr. Wang would tell me the PET scan had revealed a different form of cancer. I figured if I could have MCL without knowing it, anything was possible. I might have had stomach cancer, just like my grandfather, or something even worse. Learning our body is not as healthy as we thought tends to make us assume the worst.

Thankfully, Dr. Wang told us that his team had not found any other form of cancer in my body. They did locate the MCL on a lymph node in my left armpit and on a couple of lymph nodes in my groin. There was also a 5 percent inclusion of MCL in my bone marrow, so he labeled this stage IV MCL. They had also classified my MCL as "classic," which meant it was growing slowly and we had time to work on the perfect treatment.

We hear about stages of cancer, and stage IV sounds pretty darn terminal, but that is not the case with MCL. Stages of MCL are not tied to mortality as they are in other cancers. Stages simply let physicians know how systemically MCL has progressed.

Dr. Wang advised us against traditional treatments for my stage and type of cancer. He said that the ferocity of traditional chemotherapy and radiation treatments would inevitably lead me to leukemia, heart attacks, and other issues over the next ten years. The treatments he recommended required his team to grow stem cells in a lab, remove my bone marrow to "nuke" all the cancerous cells, put the newly grown stem cells back into my bones, and then bring me back to life. It would be brutal and put me in a very compromised position afterward.

Because most MCL patients are sixty-five or older, this comprehensive approach works fine. If a sixty-five-year-old man with cancer is kept alive until the age of seventy-five, they consider it a success. A forty-five-year-old man who passes away at fifty-five would be considered a failure.

Luckily, Dr. Wang had a much better approach to treating me. He runs the Lymphoma and Myeloma Center at MD Anderson, where, at the time, they were conducting a clinical trial for MCL treatments. He hypothesized that two immunotherapy drugs could combat MCL without the use of chemotherapy or radiation. Although he said I did not meet the criteria for phase one, he smiled and told Tina and me that phase two was opening in a couple months and I was a perfect candidate.

With this new information in hand, Tina and I drove home to wait a few months for the trial to start. My body was going to be put through a lot, and I wanted to make sure that I was strong enough to handle it. This is where the workout helped me train for treatment.

I stayed in Austin, had no symptoms besides some fatigue, and used the workout five days a week, along with bicycling two days a week. The meditation aspects of the workout helped me keep my mind clear at a time when the seriousness of the diagnosis could have caused me to spiral out of control.

During those few months, I got so strong that my mind, body and soul were all working together. Since mental health has such a strong effect on physical health, I was able to meditate myself into thinking that I was already cured of cancer and my body just needed to catch up.

CHAPTER TWO

DESIGNING THE FITFAB WORKOUT

*C*ancer is a scary word loaded uncertainty and doubt. It was not even on my radar in February of 2018 when I was designing a new weightlifting program for myself. My initial goal was simply to stop exacerbating my existing injuries and prevent new ones. I noticed that as I aged, my body started to heal much more slowly, and any injury would take me away from weightlifting for an extended period. I felt like I was walking a fine line between working out and getting injured. Something had to change in the way I approached my workouts.

When I started to think about what I needed from a weightlifting program in my forties and beyond, I knew I did not want to compromise the strength I had in my twenties. I wanted to be able to lift a sizable amount of weight without looking like an overfilled bodybuilder. I wanted a solid base of muscle; I did not care whether it was perceptible to the naked eye. Most importantly, I did not want to lose strength as I aged.

MY FIRST FORAY INTO WEIGHTLIFTING

I started weightlifting at the age of fourteen, just as I entered high school as a freshman. I vividly remember saving up to get my first bench, bar, and weights from my local Big 5 Sporting Goods in Huntington Beach, California. The weights were little more than round cement shapes of various sizes, covered in a dull copper-colored plastic. Without any formal instruction, I began like many first timers do: I spent most of my days bench-pressing and doing rudimentary curls.

Later, I signed up for football and wrestling, each of which had formal workouts designed to strengthen one's body. As a dedicated athlete in both sports, I was lifting quite often. My fellow athletes and I did not know a lot about how to properly lift weights. We would simply try to lift as much as possible. Back then, our muscles recovered quickly. There were not many lasting consequences to putting a bunch of weight on a rack and lifting it with terrible form. We just celebrated each new weight milestone.

The football and wrestling coaches helped us smooth out the rough spots of our form, and eventually we all improved. By the time I was seventeen, my weightlifting had become more accurate, the weights lifted more reasonable, and my form closer to perfect.

I wanted to build my strength outside of team workouts, so I signed up for a membership at the local gym. I met a fellow weightlifter, and we started working out together. Eventually, we became friends and exercise partners. With an accountability partner, I was lifting weights nightly, increasing the weight for each lift, and building massive amounts of clean muscle. We encouraged each other with requests for proper form and assisted with one another's last few repetitions of each exercise.

I highly recommend lifting with a partner when you are young. They are easy to find, easy to schedule, and improve outcomes. The best part is that having a friend who likes to lift weights means you can do a lot of things together.

As we get older, it is harder to find common time to work out, which is why the workout is designed to be done in solitude.

THE IMPORTANCE OF CARDIO

My work travel schedule in my midtwenties caused me to take the workouts on the road. I really had the best intention of working out in each city. At one point I was traveling to three cities per week, and while I tried to maintain my weightlifting, it slowly dropped off as I prioritized going to dinner with clients and friends in each city over exercise. My typical workout partners were two guys named Ben and Jerry from Burlington, Vermont. This was a recipe for weight gain, and I was no longer building lean muscle. I was bulking up with some intermittent workouts and plenty of Wavy Gravy ice cream.

Eventually, my travel schedule slowed down, and I looked for ways to trim my waistline.

This was when I first found enjoyment in running. At first, I would spend a couple days a week running around Austin's Lady Bird Lake on the hike-and-bike trail during my lunches. My first goal was to comfortably run a mile, then a mile and a half, then two miles, and so on.

Slowly but surely, it became my daily routine to run a three-and-one-half-mile loop. Two of my coworkers heard about my daily runs and started joining me at lunch. We worked just down the road from the hike-and-bike trail and took advantage of the showers in our office. It felt like I was finally establishing balance between my early professional career and my fitness priorities.

After running became a passion, I still lifted weights, but only occasionally. The intermittent pauses in my weightlifting schedule meant I continued to injure myself. I reached a point where running became my exercise of choice because I had not gotten injured doing it—yet. Within a couple of years, I was running ten miles per day in the scorching heat of Austin's summer when the temperature hits 104 degrees.

I had trimmed off fifty pounds of fat and muscle by the time I started training for what would have been my first marathon. As winter set in, I continued to run, with a goal of finishing the marathon in February. Given my limited stretching before and after my runs, the continual stress on my body became noticeable. My left leg's iliotibial band was being rubbed in all the wrong ways, making my daily running schedule very painful. I tried a variety of methods for running and recovery and was not able to get over the pain in my left leg.

One cold Saturday morning in February, I was on my weekly long run, which this week was going to be twenty-four miles. Around mile twenty, my left knee felt like someone was stabbing it with a rusty fork. I limped home for seven miles, nursing my iliotibial band. I was incredibly sad when I canceled my registration for the marathon. Eventually I gave up running for biking and have not gone back.

The move to biking has been great for my joints, although it lacks the amazing physical results seen during my running career. While I kept riding my bike each day, I wanted to add more weightlifting back into my workout regimen as I went into my forties. My big fear was not getting hurt; it was getting injured. Consider this real-life scenario: you are playing soccer and get kicked in the leg by another player. If you are hurt, you simply shake it off and bet back in the game. If you are injured, you are quickly removed from the game by stretcher and are diagnosed by a doctor.

WEIGHTLIFTING IN MY FORTIES

My forties greeted me with a slow metabolism and reduced testosterone. These are standard changes, but I did not expect them to change my experience at the gym. I became less of a brute and started to approach my time in the gym more passively. Despite my new outlook, I kept getting injured. I would skip days to nurse my injuries, then lose my progress and return to the gym to push myself even harder. Obviously, this just led to more injuries, and the cycle started over again and again. Something needed to change. I looked around for various workout methodologies for "retired surfers" like me and centered on a few basic ideas that, when grouped together, became the FitFAB Workout.

The Body Needs to Be Well-Hydrated

In Tom Brady's 2017 book, *The TB12 Method*, the Patriots' six-time Super Bowl champion wrote that he drinks half of his body weight in water each day during football season. He doubles the amount when exercising. For Tom, this equates to just over two gallons per day. After reading about his routine, I decided to try it myself. If it worked for an elite athlete, it was sure to improve something for me.

I knew overhydration can strip our body of essential vitamins and minerals, so I decided to start testing my body at three liters of water during my workouts. Drinking that much water throughout my workout forced me to take longer rests between sets just to get all of it down. After some trial and error, I eventually lowered my gym intake to two liters. At this level, I could ensure that I was hydrated without compromising my sleep schedule. That many bathroom breaks in the middle of the night can really ruin a good night's sleep. Best of all, I felt less soreness and pain during my weightlifting sessions.

When we work out, our body breaks down glucose into two molecules through a process called glycolysis. When our body's oxygen supply is sufficient, things work well. Under oxygen deprivation conditions, such as when we restrict our breath during a weightlifting exercise, most of the molecules are converted into lactic acid, a by-product that stays in our muscles, resulting in pain.

When our muscles use glycolysis, the lactic acid produced in the muscles' cells needs to be transported to the outside of the cells to avoid an accumulation that causes severe pain. Hydrating our body while working out allows our muscles to quickly flush the lactic acid away, helping us avoid the leading cause of pain while weightlifting.

Lactic acid tries to convince our brain we should stop lifting because our muscles hurt. But if we stop too soon, we will never get the strength results we want. Rather than trying to rewire our body's connection to the brain, it is much easier to simply add more water to our workout routines. The result is less pain, more consistent workouts, and stronger, higher-quality muscle development, all in a shorter period.

The Body Needs to Rest

Many boxers specifically train their bodies to stay strong for three minutes—the length of each round in boxing. In gyms across the world, boxers can be found pushing as hard as they can for three minutes and then resting for one minute. If they can master this rhythm during training, they know they will have the right level of endurance to face their opponents.

I never had dreams of becoming a boxer, but this cycle of work and rest intrigued me. I wanted to know more, including the benefits of intentional rest during periods of extreme training. It turns out that equal periods of training and rest help our muscles recover better. In search of anything that would help reduce pain and injury, I decided to test the cycle out at my local gym.

Over the course of a year, I varied the length of time spent lifting and resting, finally settling on two minutes for each phase. In the FitFAB Workout, we use a structure of two minutes of dedicated lifting followed by two minutes of dedicated stretching and resting.

I collected the data on how my body reacted to the varying times. Longer times felt like too much on my joints. Shorter times felt like my muscles had to stop when they were just getting started. I had friends in their forties trying out varying lengths of time too, and they reported back what they uncovered. From what my friends and I collected, two minutes is the perfect blend for muscle fatigue and recovery in those of us over forty.

The Body's Biggest Gains Can
Be Had from Negatives

Back in the early nineties, I occasionally worked out with Kimo Leopoldo at Powerhouse Gym in Huntington Beach. Kimo is a brick wall of a man. He competed in the third Ultimate Fighting Championship. This man knew his way around a gym and offered to help me with negatives on an incline bench press. When doing a negative, you spend your energy on the return motion of an exercise rather than the initial motion. For my incline bench press, this meant focusing on the weight coming down rather than going up. Kimo would help me lift the weights up and would keep me from getting hurt on the way down.

Going slow and focusing on the return meant I activated muscles that otherwise would have been resting. The result was increased strength, with a more stable muscular system that was less susceptible to injury. As we age, stability and strength become increasingly valuable for avoiding injuries and staying active into our geriatric years.

I credit Kimo for my continued focus on and enjoyment of negatives. They still work great and have been incorporated into the FitFAB Workout. Thank you, Kimo.

The Body Needs to Be in Sync
with the Brain

Weightlifting is 70 percent lifting and 30 percent believing you can lift. Whenever our brain is preoccupied with something else, our muscles will not be able to lift their maximum weight. Incorporating simple mental exercises to clear out clutter is important for learning to use that extra 30 percent of our strength.

The FitFAB Workout requires each weightlifter to be fully present when lifting. Focusing on exterior things will only lead to unrealistic decisions, poor form, poor performance, and injuries. When incorporating the meditation included later in this book, each workout will send you home with extra space in your head for positive things, including muscle recovery, because you have spent time letting go of all your negative thoughts at the gym.

The Body Needs to Be Warmed
Up like an Old Car

Imagine the whirring sounds of a forty-something-year-old car as you try to start it up. Watch yourself pump the gas to prime the carburetor and smell that whiff of stale gas as you turn the key. Turn off the ignition after hearing the motor turn a few times without igniting a spark. Pump the gas a few times and then turn the key. Blub blub blub. It hesitates and then starts up, revving with the additional gas from your foot pumping. After it starts, you gently press the gas pedal to keep it from stalling. Five minutes later, you can drive the car knowing the engine will not die on you. This, my friends, is like the body of a person over forty. Welcome to middle age. In our body's case, the warming-up process involves a lot of stretching.

Stretching is one of the biggest problems in weightlifting. Most people do not stretch nearly enough. Injuries, muscle and joint tightness, and stunted mobility are all signs that weightlifters have skipped their stretching.

Stretching is a foundation of the FitFAB Workout. We will focus on stretching just as much as on weightlifting because we cannot have the latter without the former. Stretching is not done once in our workouts, but rather it is a process we incorporate into every set and exercise.

Stretching helps bring fresh blood into our muscles, limbers them up to reduce injury, and realigns our muscle fibers to provide for increased strength.

CHAPTER THREE

THE FIVE TENETS OF THE FITFAB WORKOUT

T he FitFAB Workout is an amalgamation of research and curated advice brought together into a single unique vision for strength training. It combines decades of training experience with information gathered from the best physical therapists and sports medicine doctors.

To create the base framework for the FitFAB Workout, there first has to be a set of overarching guidelines to which we can return whenever there is a question. Consider it our workout's constitution. Its components are the guiding principles of an effective workout for anyone, but especially those of us over forty. The goal is to eliminate injuries, which gives us more time to work out and keeps us in our good habits.

The five tenets are:

1. We track minutes of weightlifting rather than number of repetitions performed.

2. We exercise slowly and with perfect form.

3. We perform positive and negative movements at the same speed.

4. We hydrate before and after every set.

5. We stagger muscle groups in a specific order.

WE TRACK MINUTES OF WEIGHTLIFTING RATHER THAN NUMBER OF REPETITIONS PERFORMED

Counting repetitions is often a bad habit left over from earlier years in the gym. Typically, it starts in high school. No matter the sport, coaches train us to think in terms of a set being ten repetitions. Why ten? It could be that it is an easy number to count, even if you are not on the dean's list. But that is not a fitness-related answer. Often, we are so desperate to get to the tenth repetition that we contort our body into all sorts of shapes to get that tenth rep completed. These contortions lead to bad form and long-term injuries—doing them after forty will not serve our body well.

Yes, counting reps is one way to track our performance, but only if each repetition is within our capabilities and done with perfect form. When we push beyond our limits, we tend to throw weights around, pushing and pulling until we can technically count it as a rep. This damages our muscles as we slip and slide, never fully in control of the weight. An uncontrolled weight transforms from a fitness tool into a hammer banging on every joint, tendon, and muscle in the primary muscle group and all the supporting muscle groups. Oftentimes, this improper form results in us injuring our backs.

Whenever I try to get ten reps, I find that I am so focused on getting the weight through the form that I forget which rep I am on. I have a hard time focusing on counting while I have a large amount of weight above my head. This was not a problem when I was younger and had a dedicated workout partner, but as I aged, the increased scheduling challenges meant I did not have someone to work out with me every time I was at the gym, so I sometimes did eleven reps, and sometimes only nine. I thought there had to be a better way, and after trial and error, I found it.

There is a better way. A simpler way. An automated way. We will use a visual timer to answer the question of "How much more do I have to go?" The key thing to remember is that we will track two minutes of weightlifting followed by two minutes of hydrating, stretching, and resting. By focusing on weightlifting until we reach a particular minute on the clock, we can get rid of the beleaguered process of counting and remembering repetitions.

Another nice thing about this method is that it gives our brain a chance to process the stress of the day without having to remember the count at the same time.

Plus, tracking minutes keeps us focused on the pureness of the movement itself. When the weight is light, we could do one rep every two seconds and go crazy to reach sixty repetitions per set. That is insane to even consider. The goal of this workout is to keep us from injury. By significantly slowing down our movements, we end up with more control of the weights. Our workouts become impactful, injury-free, and consistent—the three factors for building strength.

WE EXERCISE SLOWLY AND WITH PERFECT FORM

First-time weightlifters tend to focus on finishing a movement rather than building the muscle memory to perform it correctly. Muscle memory is like a painted lane marker on a road. It keeps us going in the right direction. Without it, we become more chaotic in our movements as the weight increases, or we feel more fatigued when performing the movements. Over time, this leads to bad habits that put us at risk of injuries as our joints take the brunt of the force and other muscles must kick in.

Even the most seemingly insignificant deviation in an exercise can lead to dire consequences. Consider squats. When we are performing a traditional squat exercise, where a barbell with weights is held in place on top of our trapezius muscles, the pair of large triangular muscles extending over our back of the neck and shoulders, it is important to keep the angle of our feet less than fifteen degrees off-center. When we flare our feet past fifteen degrees, our body loses hip function, and our femur bone rotates, which can easily tear our knees and ankles.

We do not do squats in this workout, because the only way to achieve perfect squat form is to have a coach standing next to us, moving our body to keep it in perfect alignment. It is too much to ask of anyone, so we use different exercises to obtain the same benefits as come from squats. Our knees and ankles will be much happier this way.

If you have been in a gym with younger weightlifters, you have inevitably seen people doing standing barbell curls. Often, you will see someone shrug to the side with the weight, and by lowering their shoulder and bending to the side, they look like they are throwing the barbell up rather than using their biceps, which are the target muscles, with a curl. This bending causes back muscles to flare on one side, the hips to slightly rotate out of balance, and the body to take a beating—all to take the pressure off the biceps. Not only is this dangerous, but it also reduces the biceps' range of motion.

A neon sign saying "Poor form leads you to injury and never coming back to the gym" should be plastered on every wall of the gym.

I am the first to admit that, when I was younger, I used this curling technique. It did not seem like I was hurting anything at the time. But as I got older, the injuries that had been baked into my musculoskeletal system came back to haunt me. The poor form caused pain in my sciatic nerve, which is the major nerve that branches from our lower back through our hips and buttocks and down each leg. I got bicipital tendonitis in my left arm to the point that I was unable to pick up a can of soup, let alone lift weights. It was a depressing time. I knew I had to overcome this if I was ever going to be a forty-year-old weightlifter.

After researching the various forms of tendonitis, I realized that if I could slow down when performing each exercise, I could focus on perfect form to build the right muscle memory for each movement. My left arm was unable to perform a biceps curl properly when I returned to the gym, so this was my test case for the concept.

My plan was simple: slow down to get my muscles into the right "lane," while at the same time strengthening the secondary and tertiary muscles that help the core muscle group in each exercise. The problems we create when throwing weights around can be fixed when we make proper form our top priority. As the main muscle in an exercise starts to fail, the other supporting muscles pick up the slack and keep the weight moving, thereby acting as a spotter for our main muscle group. We will not contort our body because the weight will be lighter, and we will be going slow and in control.

Muscle failure is exceptionally good. We want our muscles to fail when we lift weights. This indicates the muscle has spent all its available energy in the form of water and oxygen. Muscle failure creates opportunities for other muscles to jump in and help. This will give you the overall body strength that comes with the FitFAB Workout.

The goal of muscle failure also means we do not use traditional free weights. Instead, we use a combination of cable-and-pulley machines to eliminate any risk of injury when our muscles start to tire. If all the muscles used in a particular exercise fail, the handle of the machine will return to its starting point, and we will stop for a moment to catch our breath and replenish oxygen in our muscles. This also resets our muscles' powerband, the horizontal path the muscles' energy takes throughout a complete movement.

In exercising this way, when we reach the start of the movement, we let our muscles rest for a full two seconds before continuing the movement. This little break in the action helps reset our muscles and prevents injuries from strain that accompanies pushing or pulling a weight for an extended period.

WE PERFORM THE POSITIVE AND NEGATIVE MOVEMENTS AT THE SAME SPEED

When we visit our local gym, we likely notice people, big and small, performing exercises extremely fast. They might be pulling weights up quickly on a biceps curl and then sending their arm down just as quickly, if not more so. This is a recipe for disaster. Instead of isolating their biceps and building strength, they are forcing the muscles in their arms, shoulders, traps, wings, and lower back to work harder. The result is lower back and bicipital tendon injuries. Unfortunately, some will learn from years of this type of abuse that tendon injuries are among the more painful and debilitating ones.

The FitFAB Workout uses the slow-out/slow-in method. The first important thing to learn is how to time our breath with the first movement. For example, let's say we are performing a chest press. Our first movement is to position our hands at the sides of our chest, gripping the handles of the bar. The goal is to push the handles forward and away from our chest. When we are about to start our first movement, we take a large, slow breath in through our nose and mouth simultaneously. We then close our nose and exhale slowly through our mouth as we push the handles away from our chest. We push it very slowly for five to seven seconds. This is the positive movement, or "slow-out" portion of the movement. We call the point at which the handles are farthest from us the "apex" of the movement.

Immediately, but slowly, we change directions and start coming back from the apex. There is no resting at the apex, as this can lead to hyperextensions and other major injuries. Just like on the slow-out movement, we go slowly as we complete the slow-in motion.

Picture that we are pushing the weight forward but in an ever-decreasing manner to lower the handles. This sounds crazy, but believe me, the darn thing works. I recommend you do not consider the slow-in movement as a return to the beginning position. This would activate an entirely different set of muscles, and we want to be as focused on our chest muscles as possible.

As our handles reach the beginning position, we remove all pressure from our chest muscles by relaxing them while still holding on to the handles. The type of exercises I recommend for this workout are designed to allow us to do this one-second relaxation. Unlike a bench press, which has a small window for rest at the apex, the chest press machine has the rest at the beginning of the slow-out movement. This maximizes our muscles' powerband.

During a chest press, the muscle starts in a stretched configuration and is flexed into a tightened configuration and then stretched out again. The powerband of the chest press goes from stretched to stretched. We can visualize this through a simple chart with the time it takes to perform the movement along the x-axis and the available muscle strength along the y-axis.

This amount of available strength in a movement creates the height of our powerband. In our first repetition, the available muscle strength is remarkably high. It decreases a bit with each repetition, sometimes by a significant amount. The higher the powerband is from the zero-energy baseline, the easier it is to perform the movement (conversely, the lower the powerband, the harder the movement).

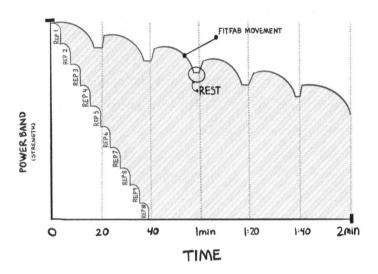

If our muscles can rest after each completed powerband, our available muscle strength is higher. The contrary is true as well; if our muscles are not allowed to rest, our available strength will be lower, and the movement harder to complete. If we continue to push as if we have a higher powerband, we risk a complete muscle failure, in which our muscle may tear or, even worse, a tendon may become inflamed or rupture.

In the slow-out/slow-in movement method, we rest for two seconds at the beginning of engaging our powerband. In our chest press example, this requires us to lower our shoulders a bit and let our arms hang on the handles. By resetting our powerband, we maintain our available muscle strength, extend our muscle to its full range, and give it a chance to get the oxygen-rich blood it needs to quickly recover before the next repetition.

You may notice that you tend to start resting for longer than two seconds as you get to the end of your two-minute set. In the chest press example, you may need to remove your hands from the handles and rotate your shoulders for a few seconds. Listen to your body, and be sure to manage your powerband for each exercise. A longer rest toward the end allows you to inhale a lot more oxygen with each breath.

We should strive for a powerband with a slow seven-to-ten-second outward movement and a ten-second inward movement, followed by a two-second rest period. You will probably fluctuate, tending toward shorter intervals as your muscles start to fatigue. It is not critical to be at the ten-second mark. It is more of an aspiration than a rule.

The beauty of the slow-out/slow-in method is that it aligns our incentives with each exercise. Rather than performing ten quick repetitions per set, we perform two minutes of intense power-bands with varying rest periods. By reducing the number of repetitions during our set, we increase our strength tremendously.

I saw the proof one evening when a friend and I went to the gym while on vacation. He and I are of similar build and what appears to be similar muscle mass. We talked about what weight we each normally used for the chest press. It turned out we were only a few pounds different, so we chose the lower weight. I started my first set with a perfectly executed slow-out/slow-in movement and kept going for two minutes. My friend was intrigued by it and decided to start using the same method.

It was around the one-minute mark when he asked me, "How many seconds do I have left?" He could barely talk from the breath he was holding. When I told him sixty seconds were left, the look on his face was one of pure defeat. He was not going to make it to two minutes, not even close. My strength had dwarfed his because he was used to an extremely fast ten repetitions, which may or may not have been done with perfect form. He thought it was going to be the same when he used the two-minute slow-out/slow-in method. While we had a similar max chest press weight, his chest's powerband height was much lower than mine.

WE HYDRATE BEFORE AND
AFTER EVERY SET

Adequate hydration is an essential success factor of the FitFAB Workout. Proper water intake helps our body move lactic acid and other nutrients around our muscles. It is not enough to occasionally take a sip from a water fountain at the gym. Our adult bodies are 60 percent water. Muscles are 79 percent water. If that percentage drops by too much, we can experience various ailments, including significant muscle tears, which lead to large gaps in our training and little to no progress at the gym.

Back injuries, which are also common when we work out dehydrated, are some of the worst because our back is central to everything we do. Our back is a set of bones separated by discs to keep them from rubbing together. These discs between each of the spinal column bones are soft, jelly-like pads that protect our backbones from injury. Together, they act like a cushion for our spines, and when we become dehydrated, they can lose their cushioning effect. The result is significant pain throughout our back and neck.

If we are feeling thirsty during our workout, it is too late. Our body has already suffered from dehydration. To help prevent this, I designed the FitFAB Workout to include hydration steps along the way. Each step includes time to drink water and allow our body to recover in real time. The goal is longevity and sustainability. For the routine to work for us, we must take each step seriously.

Keep in mind that we can also drink too much water. During my trial-and-error period of building this workout, I would drink three-quarters of a gallon of water when I was at the gym. This turned out to be too much. One half gallon is the perfect amount for the exercises we are performing.

You will find a water bottle in the equipment section of this book that should work well for the length of time we will spend at the gym. I recommend filling it halfway with ice cubes before you head to the gym, as there is nothing better than refreshing our body with cold water when working out. It is critical to drink water before and after each set. Those few sips will do wonders to keep our body performing.

Some people like to sweeten their water with zero-calorie, artificially sweetened drink mixes. But I do not recommend putting anything in the bottle except water and ice. Our body needs water to perform. Anything we add may interfere with its ability to quickly absorb the water. This entire fitness philosophy is based around doing what our body needs for long-lasting health, so skip the sweeteners.

WE STAGGER MUSCLE GROUPS
IN A SPECIFIC ORDER

Our muscles need time to rest after we put pressure on them. Performing the same exercise every day will lead to injuries from overuse, so we will stagger our workout over several days.

Day 1 will be focused on our chest muscles. The next day, we will work on our back. The days following will be legs, arms, and then shoulders. By staggering the muscle groups in this way, we give each group a chance to fully recover. They will be the primary focus on their day of the week, and they will get lightly used through secondary and tertiary movements on the other days.

We will also perform the different workouts in complementary ways. The first day is always chest. Our chest workout will also work our triceps. Our triceps will feel the workout, but our chest is the primary muscle group for that day.

When I was younger, I loved trying new workout techniques, and I started working my back and biceps muscles together. What I found was that if I did not work my triceps in the same workout, I would go to sleep and wake up with my arms unable to fully extend. This was painful, and, on several occasions, I had to run to the gym and do a few triceps exercises to relieve my biceps so I could fully extend my arms. But alas, it was usually too late by then, and I had to spend most of the day in pain.

We will order our workouts so that the day after chest exercises is back exercises. The two are complementary, so when we work one and then the other, we maintain a sense of balance. We will also work our biceps and triceps on the same day. This will allow us to have two days of secondary arm exercises, followed by a day of primary arm exercises.

We will end our five days of lifting for the week with a shoulder workout. There are several reasons for this. First, our shoulders get a secondary workout on each of the previous days' exercises except for legs, so by the time we get to them, they are already partially fatigued. If we were to start out the week working our shoulders, we would have a harder time performing the chest, back, and arm workouts.

Second, if we were to perform our shoulder workouts first, we would be in shoulder pain for each subsequent day because our shoulder muscles would not be resting enough. By leaving shoulders to the last day, we give them the most recovery time, given that they are so crucial to exercising the other muscle groups.

Last, if you ever need to skip a day, I recommend skipping shoulders, as they will have already received a lot of training on each of the previous days. This does not mean we should not do shoulders. It just means that we should not feel bad skipping shoulder day if we must cut our week short (unlike skipping leg day, which is a no-no).

To recap, here is the schedule we will use.

Day 1	Day 2	Day 3	Day 4	Day 5	Day 6	Day 7
Chest	Back	Legs	Arms	Shoulders	Rest	Rest

Notice that this schedule leaves two days with no weight training at all. This is the important time needed to let our muscles and joints rest and heal. To achieve our goals, we need to approach rest with the same dedication with which we approach strength exercises. The healing process is critical to reducing joint inflammation, which typically leads to arthritis and severe pain.

Chest muscles get a full seven-day rest period as a primary muscle group. They get a four-day rest period as a secondary muscle group because our chest will be used as a helper muscle when we work our arms. They will get a three-day rest as a tertiary muscle group when we work our shoulders. The same applies to all other muscle groups.

The FitFAB Workout focuses on training to the point of muscle failure. Muscle failure is different from muscle injury. While we may not experience muscle failure in the first few months of training, we will eventually experience it. At the point of muscle failure, secondary muscle groups kick in and help our primary muscles finish the movement.

CHAPTER FOUR

TWO MINUTES

The FitFAB Workout is a program for our mind as much as our body because by reducing our body's cortisol levels, we help our body maintain its weight. The workout is divided into two-minute blocks. I have found that going over two minutes has a negative effect on our body, and we reach a point around the three-minute mark at which our body is unable to withstand the pressure and inevitably reaches the point of injury. Two minutes balances the fatigue and muscle failure of a good workout with increased muscle strength to reach the muscle maximization coefficient as described below. These two minutes will be the most valuable, and at times the hardest, of our day.

MUSCLE MAXIMIZATION COEFFICIENT

This term refers to the total available strength our muscles can withstand prior to failing. When we go way past the two-minute mark on a set, we run the risk of a catastrophic muscle collapse, which can lead to major injuries. These injuries can, and oftentimes do, completely stop our training. Among possible injuries are sprains that stretch or tear our ligaments, the bands of fibrous tissue connecting bones to bones at joints. Another potential injury is a muscle strain that stretches or tears our muscles or tendons. Since our tendons link muscles to bones, it can be quite painful for them to stretch, tear, or swell. In some cases, they can even pull bones apart, which can lead to permanent damage.

Unlike our muscles, which can repair themselves with more muscle tissue, our tendons are replaced with the formation of scar tissue with extraordinarily little regenerative capability. Too much scar tissue can force us to get costly and painful medical procedures to replace tendons.

MANAGING OUR EGO

There are going to be other people working out at the gym while we are there. The other members in the gym can trigger our reptilian brains into posturing. You will find yourself wanting to impress others with bigger weights and faster reps. Avoid these urges at all costs. Remember, our goal is overall fitness and strength, not building mass. We want to thrive in our older years, and we will not be able to do that if we make ego-driven mistakes in the gym. To keep on track with our workout, show up five days a week, show up every week, and eventually we will be stronger and fitter than ever before.

Think of the gym like high school. People are so worried about what they look like to others that they often forget the fundamentals. We can reverse this thinking by asking ourselves how many seconds per hour at the gym we look at other people. It is normally just a few seconds here and there. This is the exact amount of time people are looking at us. They are not watching our every move, nor how much weight we are lifting. They will stare if we injure ourselves because nobody can take their eyes off a person whose shoulder is dislocated. Trust me; I dislocated my shoulder when I was in my early twenties, and it was a spectacle.

Egos get involved in almost every sport we tackle. When I shifted from being a weightlifter to a runner, I was embarrassed, as I ran slowly and over short distances. I had the thought of trying to find time when nobody was around and eventually had to come to grips with the fact that everyone was out running to improve themselves. They were probably just as worried as I was. Not until a couple years into running would I run without a shirt on when it was hot out.

Ego is something we all wrestle with at the gym. This is one of the reasons I like to close my eyes during the two minutes. It removes the distraction of people looking at me as I lift. Consider closing your eyes to focus on the movement and remove the distractions.

GOING IT ALONE

The FitFAB Workout is a self-journey. You are in competition with only yourself. There is no need to include others when you work out. You are there to clear your mind, focus on your health, and get a good workout. In that order. Without your head in the game, your workouts will be less productive, as we can lose up to 30 percent of our strength when our head is not fully committed.

We will inevitably come to the gym with a lot of stressors racing through our mind, but we can leave the gym feeling peaceful, energized, and positive. I remember the night I was at the gym after hearing about my stage IV cancer diagnosis. I sat there on the pectoral fly machine sobbing. Closing my eyes, I placed the back of my thumbs against my eyebrows and gave myself permission to stop thinking about what this would mean to my family. It helped me get back to preparing my body for the fight.

The mental benefits of the FitFAB Workout cannot be overstated. Five days a week, we dedicate ourselves to a period in which we can relieve our brain of stressors, engage our body, and grow stronger. The mind portion of the workout will help us categorize and structure our stressors in a way that enables us to perform at a high level.

Another thing I have noticed is that a clear mind will not give up. The idea of cutting the workout short and going home will be less appealing once we have cleared out the clutter. There is nobody keeping us at the gym besides ourselves. This intrinsic motivation teeters precariously with our mood. Therefore, we focus on clearing our head. It aligns with our overall incentives around fitness and strength.

CHAPTER FIVE

RECOVERING AT THE GYM FROM A HOSPITAL STAY

After a dinner out, I was driving my family home from an ice cream shop ten blocks from our house. My body felt a little weird, so I opened my phone's heart rate monitor app and put the phone in its cradle on the dashboard. The initial reading told me that my heart rate was approximately eighty-five beats per minute.

A moment later, my wife and I watched as the heart rate quickly spiked. I only glanced over from time to time, and in two minutes it had spiked to 125. Rather than risk driving the final two blocks to our house, I pulled the car over, put it into park, turned on the hazard lights, and asked my wife to call 911.

As she called, I started to feel intense pressure in my temples. I felt very sweaty and opened the door to get some fresh air. The last thing I saw as I left the car was my heart rate reaching 158.

I stood up to feel the pressure in my head bubble up, and I collapsed, falling to the ground. Thankfully, a friendly neighbor was driving by and saw our car with its hazard lights on. I collapsed into her arms as she came over to see if everything was okay, saving me from a head injury.

I was unconscious for fifteen seconds, and when I awoke, I was looking at my wife and our neighbor. The paramedics arrived, by which time I was back in the driver's seat, catching my breath and trying to get my bearings. I was confused and worried.

Our five-year-old son did not fully understand the severity of the situation, but our eight-year-old was very upset. I remember seeing the tears in his eyes as he watched me get into the ambulance. The paramedics had me sit down, and they put electrocardiogram leads on my chest and legs. They watched my heart rate drop to thirty-six beats per minute, and I collapsed. Something had cut off the blood supply, and my body essentially rebooted itself.

I asked for my wife to come into the ambulance, and I immediately kissed her and held her hand. My body was very cold, and my legs were shivering as shock took effect. Fear was coursing through my body. The stressors of life vanished in an instant, and at that moment, I was only worried about getting to the hospital and surviving.

I was worried about keeping my heart going as the doctors performed test after test. Everything came back looking normal. The doctors said I looked healthy. My electrocardiogram monitor showed a clean heart rate and consistent heartbeat. I was discharged home after a final CAT scan showed I was clear of any risk.

It turned out the episode had been the result of stressors from my work as an entrepreneur. Each doctor I spoke to explained that stress can do a number on the body, and it had created a situation in which my brain had to reboot—twice.

This episode caused me to lose a bit of strength. Going back to my FitFAB Workout, I decreased the weight I lifted in each exercise by 25 percent. It was important for me to recover fully and maintain my overall health. With so many unexpected obstacles coming my way, I was not going to let my ego create more health issues. I reduced my weights and built my strength back slow and steady.

I tell this story to show that we will all inevitably have something happen that forces us to stop our routine. In these moments, our basic instincts tell us to go back to the gym and push ourselves. We need to prove that we are still young, strong, and healthy. But overexerting ourselves will never prove that. This is our ego again wanting to get in the way. In fact, overexertion will make our recovery longer and more difficult. Instead, be smart about restarting your workout routine. Lower your weights by 25 percent. If you have been away from the gym for more than a month, as many were during the COVID-19 pandemic in 2020, drop your weights by 50 percent. Fitness and strength are not destinations; they are journeys we embark on for ourselves.

Whether it is cancer, COVID-19, or even a fluttering heart rate, the FitFAB Workout can be easily adjusted to fit any situation. If we follow the routine, we will get the strength results we want and the long-term fitness we need.

CHAPTER SIX

FIGURING OUT HOW MUCH TO LIFT

One of the largest struggles people that are new to the gym have is identifying how much weight to lift at the beginning. Too little and they will not see the progress they envision; too much and they will become very sore, avoiding the gym for a full week as they recover.

To eliminate any confusion, everyone starts every exercise in the FitFAB Workout with just five pounds. There is no doubt we will be able to lift five pounds, but we must go slow and build the muscles that support the main muscles we are working. We are more focused on form at this point than how much weight we can lift. Weight will come later. I will never ask you to do something I have not done myself. By starting at five pounds, we will crush any problems with our ego as we focus on perfect form.

From there, each week we get to make one choice per exercise: keep it at the same weight or move it up by five pounds. Resist the temptation to start at a higher weight. Increasing the weights slowly will, in turn, build up the supporting muscle groups for each exercise over time.

We know we are ready to increase the weight for an exercise by five pounds when we can handle the new weight for two minutes. We will find that moving the weights up each week will cause us to quickly reach a plateau where the weight seems like our maximum. But it is not. It is just a weight at which we need to stay for more than one week. I have had plateaus last four or five weeks because the weight was one my supporting muscles needed time to get used to. After a few weeks of training at the same weight, I was able to push past the plateaus. I know you will be able to do the same.

There is one change to these rules, which goes into effect after we reach twenty-five pounds for any given exercise. On that exercise, we will do our first set using half the weight. This is to let our muscles get used to the movements, as starting out with a massive weight can cause an injury.

Within a short period of time, we will be lifting a lot of weight. By moving by five pounds each week, we can go from five to one hundred pounds in just four and a half months. Since this workout is a journey rather than a destination, our strength will continue to build without us suffering exercise-limiting injuries. We will find it funny that, at one time, we thought ten pounds was heavy, and now we are lifting fifty pounds.

CHAPTER SEVEN

HOW
TO
LIFT

F ree weights create a lot of problems for people new to the gym. They will walk over and grab dumbbells and start lifting them. Their form will be poor, and they will suffer micro-injuries from small tears that occur when improper form is coupled with an improper weight.

To avoid such complications, the FitFAB Workout only uses cable-and-lever-based exercises. Since we do not count repetitions, we are not worried about squeezing out the last few reps with poor form. We only count time. Those two focused minutes.

Our first two minutes are for drinking water, stretching, and mentally preparing using the meditation in Chapter 11 to clear our mind of stressors. Then the fun begins: lifting.

For every exercise except for abdominal exercises, we will go slowly. I mean slowly! Let's say we are doing a pushing exercise like a lever-based chest press. We will push the handles up for about five to seven seconds, and then once we reach the top, we will pause for a half second, then slowly lower the bar. This reverse direction should take us ten to fifteen seconds. The total time for one full rep should be about fifteen to twenty seconds.

When we get to the bottom of the stroke, we will rest for one full second, which will also give us a chance to get a full breath, and then we will start pushing back up slowly. Slow and steady movements build those supporting muscles, which are key to reaching our full potential.

There will be times when we will be near the end of our two-minute set and we will not be able to get the weight all the way to the top of the movement. When this happens, go as far as you can, and continue slowly bringing it down. Do this until the end of the set, keeping in mind that you may only be moving the weight a small percentage of the distance. This will build those supporting muscles as well.

For every exercise, we tighten our abdominal muscles so that we continue to strengthen our core while we work out our other muscles.

BREATHING

Normally in weightlifting, a person will take a deep breath and push the air out as they lift. While this works well for traditional weightlifting, we will be using our breath a bit differently. We need to keep breathing through the motions since this is about time and not repetitions. The first push/pull/lift will probably feel more akin to traditional weightlifting, but as we get past the first few inches and slow down, our breath will run out. My preference is to breathe in through my nose and out through my mouth. It is important we do not feel out of breath in the middle of our two minutes, because that means we do not have enough oxygen for our muscles. Keep breathing throughout each set.

RESTING

Resting at the gym is just as important as lifting. Once we finish a set, we will take two minutes to drink water, stretch, massage the muscles we are using, and recover. Our body needs this time to move fresh oxygen to the muscle groups we stretch. Here are the things to do with our two minutes of rest.

Drink

In the first few seconds after we finish an exercise, we grab our water bottle and drink about four to five big sips of water. This will keep our muscles lubricated, so they do not cramp or lose power. You will get used to the pace of drinking water during the workout. The key thing is that you will never feel thirsty.

Stretch

After we finish our water, we let our body remain stationary for five to ten seconds. This lets the water pass the esophagus and reach the stomach. This brief period also reduces the chance of the water coming back up when we stretch.

Each exercise has its own stretching technique. Follow the stretching guidelines for each exercise. We stretch for twenty seconds on each side, which warms up any cold muscles and straightens muscle fibers that may have healed in a shortened or spaghetti-style manner. Stretching also allows our muscle fibers to elongate by reducing the overlap between thin and thick myofilament sets in the healing process.

Massage

The key to getting the water to the right places is to move a muscle around using personal sports massage. We take the pressure off our muscles by rubbing them and moving them around. Massage each muscle for twenty seconds. Begin by pressing deep into the muscle with your fingers. Vigorously move it around to get rid of any lactic acid that may have built up. Slowly lighten up the pressure and jiggle the muscle with your fingers to loosen it. It may take a few times to get it exactly right. This is another opportunity to experiment and see what works best for your muscles.

Recover

After your muscle massage, get situated on the machine, close your eyes, and use the mental workout from Chapter 11 to remove any stressors that may still be plaguing your workout. As you get ready to start a new set, let all the air out of your lungs and slowly take in your first big breath. Imagine your heart is slowing down so it can prepare for the next two minutes. Keep an eye on the clock and as it counts down to the start of the two minutes, and begin lifting.

WHAT TO DO BETWEEN EXERCISES

There will be a natural gap between exercises in which we will need to wipe down the equipment and move to the next machine. There are a few things we need to keep track of when moving from one exercise to the next.

First, make sure you have enough water to get you through your next exercise. The worst thing is to begin your rest period without enough water. If you do not have enough to make it through the next exercise, stop the clock and go fill your water bottle. Start the clock when you get to your next machine.

If someone else is using your next machine, stop the clock and wait patiently. Consider sitting on the floor with your eyes closed and doing some deep breathing to help oxygenate your blood (and, in turn, your muscles). Maybe even continue the mental workout from Chapter 11. If the wait becomes too long, simply move to another exercise and come back to this one later. Just make sure not to do two straight exercises that focus on the same primary muscle. For example, when working our arms, we are going to work our biceps and then our triceps. We can start with triceps if all biceps machines are busy, but try to start with biceps, as a rule of thumb.

CHAPTER EIGHT

PAIN

P ain is an interesting subject because in weightlifting, it comes in two flavors: sore and injured. It is important to know how to identify these and how each will affect our workout regimen.

SORE VERSUS INJURED

Feeling sore after a workout is good. We strive to be sore. It means that our body is being pushed. Because we start with five pounds in the beginning, do not expect to feel sore in the early workouts. Soreness will come over time and will be mitigated by water intake, stretching, and meditation. Yes, meditation can help reduce soreness. The simple act of training our brain to focus on things besides our sore muscles will affect how we feel during and after each workout. Your mind is a powerful tool and should be used at each stage of the FitFAB Workout.

Muscle fatigue, the healing of previous injuries, or even the way we sit at our desks each day can cause soreness. We will inevitably take our sore body into the gym. The most important thing we will want to recognize each time we are at the gym is when that bit of soreness turns into an injury.

As we say in our family when we play sports, if you are injured, we must take you to the doctor to help heal your injuries. If you are just sore, you can get back in the game.

I used to work out in the dumbest way when I was younger. Feeling invincible, I overworked my biceps because they were growing rapidly. Sadly, I did not realize it until it was too late that my mistakes had caused bicipital tendonitis. My left arm had acute pain that got worse with each repetition. It finally caused me to stop a curl mid-movement. The pain was unbearable, and by the time I had stopped, my biceps had gone beyond failure to injury. I could barely lift a can of soup. It felt permanent. I stopped lifting and went on to other sports.

The tendonitis came back when I started weightlifting in my forties. What I did to fix the injury has worked on several other injuries over the years, including lower back injuries. Trust that we have a way to work out while we heal ourselves.

DIAGNOSING AN INJURY

The moment you feel acute pain, stop the workout. Make a note that the exercise caused pain, and move on to the next. Stop any additional exercises that cause pain, flag them like the first, and continue to the next exercise. We may get to the end of the workout without being able to complete any exercise, which means we determined that all exercises for that muscle group cause injury. This is a success because we gathered good data about our body.

The following week, we cut all weights in half for the exercises we flagged as painful. If our pain comes back at the new level, stop the exercise, flag it for injury again, and move on to the next. If this happens two weeks in a row, take a week off from working out and fix the injury.

FIXING AN INJURY

In the equipment section of this book, I suggest investing in a red-light-therapy flashlight. This tool is invaluable. When you get back home from the gym, apply the red light to the injured area, making sure to move the light to different positions after each minute. Repeat this three to four times daily for five days.

When we return to the gym, we cut our weights in half one last time. We are going to strengthen our muscles by fixing the injury with lighter weight, taking care to not increase weight too fast and to let our body heal. Listen to your body as it tells you whether you are lifting too much. Your body is your map, and I am your Sherpa, leading you on the journey. Our muscles will heal, and any tendonitis will resolve with the red-light therapy and plenty of rest.

The key to the FitFAB Workout is to reduce the chances of getting injured. Sometimes injuries are due to circumstances outside of the gym, such as a fall. We will uncover the muscles that need major work through this workout. The ones needing the most help will make themselves known and they will, in turn, get stronger through the process. This is not a race. It is a way of working out. Trust the process.

CHAPTER NINE

POST-WORKOUT RECOVERY

Y ou have read a lot about what to do at the gym, but what we do outside of the gym is just as important long-term. Without proper recovery techniques, we will injure ourselves and lose any initial progress we may have found.

Thirty-five minutes to one hour on each of the five exercise days will be spent working out. That leaves twenty-three hours to heal during those days. Those can make or break the gains from the gym. If we do not take care of our body outside of the gym, all the working out in the world will not help us.

This was never clearer than when I was working out in between countless cancer treatments in Houston. My oncologist had me on numerous medications, which took a toll on my body. Working out allowed me to process the medications quickly, and I believe it is one of the reasons I had no side effects from the medications. I was taking incredibly good care of my body during those elusive twenty-three hours after the workouts.

Follow these steps as you leave the gym.

TAKE A PICTURE OF YOURSELF

After you complete a workout and before you leave the gym, take a picture of yourself in the mirror. Your muscles will be pumped up, and it will help you create a photo diary of your progress. Make each photo a head-to-toe picture in the same mirror. Stand the same way each time so you can see the changes. I have been doing this for years, and I can find a picture from a few days ago and compare it to a picture from a year or two ago. The changes are noticeable across larger chunks of time, but it is impossible to know how much you have changed without physical evidence. Remember, we are not looking for immediate improvement but for constant improvement over time.

REPLENISH YOUR ELECTROLYTES

Because we dedicated time throughout our workout to drinking water, we will not need a bunch of water immediately after our workout. But we will still need electrolytes to replenish our body and help us recover. Immediately after your workout, pick up an electrolyte-filled drink (stay away from high-calorie ones, which will undo your hard work). This step is easy, especially if you carry electrolyte packets so you can refill your water bottle at the gym and mix the drink before you leave.

Electrolytes help balance the amount of water in our body and its acid/base (pH) level. They also help move nutrients into our cells and waste out of our cells. Alternatively, we can eat foods rich in electrolytes, such as avocados, bananas, beans, oranges, potatoes, spinach, strawberries, and turkey.

REST

Resting after working out is just as important as lifting. My preference is to work out late in the evening, so the only thing left to do when I get home is cool down and go to sleep. The healing power of sleep accelerates the recovery in our muscles, and since we are trying to push our muscles to their safe optimum performance with an ever-increasing powerband, rest is a most important step.

If you work out in the morning, be sure to rest throughout the day. If your job requires a lot of sitting, and after the gym you go back to the office, realize that your body is recovering and your muscles starting to heal in a seated position, which may make it tougher to stand up later. Be sure to stretch once an hour for the first three hours after working out in the morning.

Our muscles will get a rest each week by virtue of our staggered approach to working muscle groups. At the end of each week, we will be left with two days to rest without lifting. Choose a method of resting by keeping in mind that you will be back at the gym for a chest workout in just a few days.

It does not matter what you do on these two days of rest if you are not at the gym. I have ridden my bicycle, swum, and even walked long distances. The key is not putting weight on the muscles.

CHAPTER TEN

THE EQUIPMENT

There have been countless pieces of equipment presented to me from various companies over the course of my weightlifting career. The problem with wraps, belts, and other tools is that they are cumbersome to carry around the gym. I used to carry a big bag of equipment to the gym. It was ridiculous and unnecessary for the FitFAB Workout. I have selected the following equipment specifically to make weightlifting enjoyable and successful, without requiring us to carry around that huge bag.

GLOVES

One of the reasons some people do not lift weights is that they get calluses on their palms and fingers. Blistered hands and stiff calluses can significantly impact our daily lives. I write software for a living, and that means I need to be able to type quickly and effortlessly, without any hand injuries. We can eliminate all these issues with the use of properly fitting gloves.

Gloves are used for two things: keeping our hands blister- and callus-free and supporting our wrists on the exercises where they can become fatigued before our muscles. This workout is not about building a strong grip; it is about building a strong body. If we only increased weight as our grip could handle it, we would not get very far.

I recommend Harbinger's Pro Wristwrap weightlifting gloves with the vented and cushioned leather palm area. The palm vents help remove the sweat that can cause gloves to slip around on our hands and create blisters and sore spots. The key thing is to pick the right-sized glove. It should not slip around your hand when you are holding a weight, nor should it be uncomfortably tight.

Gloves tend to loosen over time due to moisture in the leather, which makes them become ineffective at protecting our hands. The integrated wrist strap on Harbinger's Pro Wristwrap gloves allows us to reset each glove's position between sets. I tend to tighten the gloves prior to each set and loosen them between sets to let my hands and wrists recover.

LIFTING HOOKS

Gloves help protect our hands when we are performing pushing exercises. With only four fingers pulling, even small weights can challenge our grips during a two-minute set. While gloves help a little with exercises that require us to grip a bar or handle and pull it toward our body, as well as reducing or eliminating blisters, lifting hooks help even more. These are foam-covered straps that wrap around our wrists and connect to plastic-coated hooks that allow us to pull weight toward our body without relying solely on our grip strength. Without lifting hooks, our grip can fatigue up to three times as quickly as our muscles, and grip strengths vary more widely between people than muscle strength.

Pulling a bar or handle for two minutes without help will fatigue your fingers, wrists, and forearms long before your back, shoulder, or arm muscles. The hook portion of the lifting hook is clipped over the bar or handle when we perform pulling exercises using such equipment as the row, pull-down, cable row, or even cable shrugs machine.

These hooks will seem like overkill when you first put them on, but just wait until your first set. The soft foam core comforts our wrists while our four fingers comfortably wrap over the hook, dramatically increasing the amount of weight we can pull.

If you are wondering why I went with lifting hooks instead of straps, I have used cloth lifting straps, foam-padded lifting straps, and other variations on the theme and found each of them caused a tugging sensation, as though my hand wanted to separate from my arm at the wrist. I took the leap of faith with lifting hooks and have never looked back.

WATER BOTTLE

Most gyms have a water fountain, but taking repeated trips there is burdensome when we only have two minutes between sets and exercises.

Before every set, we will drink three to four big sips, equating to just over three ounces of water. We need to build a habit of carrying water with us in a large water bottle. Without it, we are guaranteed to dehydrate.

We calculate our water consumption using a simple formula. We drink three ounces of water for each of three sets for each of four exercises. This equates to thirty-six ounces of water per workout, or just over a liter of water.

Thankfully, we can use a forty-ounce water bottle to make life easy. See-through bottles are great because we can keep track of how much water we have left.

I use a forty-ounce Contigo AutoSpout because it has a foldable rubber spout that prevents contaminants from getting into or on the mouthpiece of the bottle. This is especially important after the COVID-19 pandemic, as many gyms have closed public watering areas.

Make sure to get a bottle that is dishwasher safe because we want to wash it regularly. If your water bottle ever starts to smell, just add one tablespoon of bleach to four ounces of water, shake vigorously for three minutes, rinse thoroughly with fresh water, and let the bottle air-dry.

SPEAKER CLOCK APP

A key component of the FitFAB Workout is the two-minute set. Most cell phones will go dark after one minute when they are not being used, which means we cannot easily use our phones without an application that stays open for the full two minutes.

My recommendation is to use a speaker clock application for timing since we are not counting reps. I have one with big, bold numbers that are easy to see from a distance, which is good because the phone may be a few feet in front of us, depending on the exercise we are performing.

WIRELESS NOISE-CANCELING HEADPHONES

I find it extremely helpful to reduce the noise of the gym by using noise-canceling headphones connected to my cell phone via Bluetooth. The lack of wires makes working out much easier, especially as we focus on the slow movements the FitFAB Workout requires.

RED-LIGHT THERAPY

Our tendons and ligaments rarely get a large supply of fresh blood. This means they are slower to heal and, therefore, vulnerable during the workout and recovery phases. Red-light therapy can quickly increase the blood flow to joints and muscles while also reducing pain.

To use the red light, press and hold the light against your skin nearest the joint or muscle to which you want to apply the therapy. Let the light sit on your skin for a minute. Turn off the light if it does not automatically turn off after a minute. Move the light to another position on the joint and repeat. Three minutes of red-light therapy is enough to stimulate new blood flow. Consider applying the light prior to going to the gym and then reapplying after the workout and the next day.

Note: be careful to never stare at the red light, as it can harm our eyes.

CHAPTER ELEVEN

THE FITFAB MENTAL WORKOUT

One of the biggest benefits of the FitFAB Workout is the mental clarity and focus we get from managing the stressors we bring to the gym. As we grow older, more stressors impact our daily lives. For me, those stressors went beyond the standard family and career anxieties; I was also navigating stage IV cancer treatment. While my time at the gym was certainly about making myself as healthy as possible as I moved through treatments, it was also about having space to clear my mind. Mental focus was just as important as physical health to overcoming the obstacles in my path. I came up with a meditation that helped me clear my mind, and I encourage you to incorporate it into your workout.

This meditation is about clearing our mind to allow it to fully engage in our lift. We will categorize our stressors into three distinct groups: things from the past, things in the present, and things coming up in the future.

We start by turning on our background music to drown out the noise from the gym. With the noise-canceling headphones in place we should be able to focus our mind on the meditation and then the workout. Next, we close our eyes to begin our meditation.

Next, we listen to the things going through our head. As the first stressor pops into focus, we want to immediately evaluate it. If it is in the past, we whisper to ourselves, "I give myself permission to not worry about [the stressor] anymore." We know we cannot change the past, and this verbal reminder cues our brain to let the thought go.

If our stressor involves a future event, we determine whether it is on our calendar. If it is not, we stop the workout and put it on our calendar to worry about later. I want you to put things on your calendar with the title "Worry about [the stressor]," as this allows our brain to let go of the worry. We can schedule the time to worry about the stressor right after our workout, tomorrow, or sometime in the future. We want our brain to know the stressor has been tracked and we will worry about it when the calendar says to. Then we go back to our meditation, close our eyes, and whisper to ourselves, "I give myself permission to not worry about [the stressor] anymore." It is important for us to act right away so that the thought can leave our mind as soon as possible.

If the issue we are worrying about is something in the present, we must ask ourselves, "Is this something that will simply go into the past if I do nothing about it?" If the answer is yes, we verbally give ourselves permission to let it go and move on to the next worry.

But what if the issue we are worrying about is something we must address right now? For example, one evening I had a difficult conversation with my wife, Tina, prior to going to the gym. She was headed to bed soon, but the topic was unresolved, so I stopped the workout, went home, resolved the issue with her, and then returned to the gym to finish my workout.

You heard that right. We stop and go address it right now. This is better than sitting there at the gym, stewing about something we cannot get out of our head.

Now that we have cleared our mind, it is time to apply that mental strength to our workout. We start by visualizing the muscles we are working. We feel minor pain as our muscles stretch and contract under strain. Small pains are to be expected, and we cannot ignore them. We can again use the verbal cue "I give myself permission not to worry about that small pain in my [muscle]."

We repeat this process until there is nothing bothering us. Clearing our mind and completely focusing on our workout takes a bit of practice. But soon we will have trained ourselves to let go of thoughts before they interrupt our focus. Our mind and body will know that inside the gym, we are focusing on fitness and health. Nothing else matters.

We want to pay attention to any significant pain that may indicate an injury. It takes a bit of practice, and over time, we will be able to intentionally turn off pain receptors in our body. This is important, as pain is something we are all hyperaware of. However, we are at the gym, lifting weights. Mild pain is to be expected. We want to turn off our pain receptors for the mild pain and only worry when things really hurt.

CHAPTER TWELVE

THE FITFAB BODY WORKOUT

T he body portion of the FitFAB Workout is designed to strengthen the major muscle groups in our body while simultaneously building supporting muscles. We are going to be lifting very slowly. We may not sweat very much because the goal here is to keep our heart rate low.

We will be working out one body-part group per day, and each group will be the focus of one day per week. The goal is to give our joints and muscles ample time to recover. Each muscle group will get four to five exercises. There will also be an extra core exercise since our core can be worked out every day.

This is what each week will look like. It does not matter which day of the week you start the cycle on, but stick to the same starting day each week.

Day 1: Chest

Day 2: Back

Day 3: Legs

Day 4: Arms

Day 5: Shoulders

Day 6: Rest

Day 7: Rest

Do not mix up the order. We want to allow for proper rest periods each week. We are working complementary muscle groups, which is key to protecting our body from injury.

RECOMMENDED EXERCISES

I have created a list of exercises you can do at most gyms. The FitFAB Workout works exclusively with cable-and-lever machines to prevent injury and focus on building consistent strength. Free weights can move in any direction and therefore present too many variables to be helpful for weightlifters over forty. Each cable-and-lever machine restricts our body to a specific path.

Day 1: Chest

Our chest comprises two distinct muscle groups, referred to together as the pectorals or "pecs." The pectoralis minor connects our rib cage to the area just under our collarbone by our shoulder. It is used to spread the shoulder blades when contracted and bring them together when expanded.

The pectoralis major consists of a small area connected below our collarbone and extending in front of and below our shoulder muscles. We use this muscle to raise our upper arm.

The larger area connects the center of our sternum to the same area in front of and below our shoulder muscles. We use these muscles to bring our arm toward our body's midline. They also help us rotate our upper arm.

Make sure to select at least one abdominal exercise to go with the chest workout, so we keep building our core each day.

The following chest exercises are performed wearing gloves, so we will only need to bring our water bottle and gloves for Day 1 exercises.

Exercise 1: Lower-Pivot Chest Press Machine

The chest press with the lower pivot point simulates a bench press and, as such, strengthens our pectoralis major muscles. The seated position allows us to feel comfortable, while the split handles eliminate any chance that the machine will put direct pressure on our chest and cause injury.

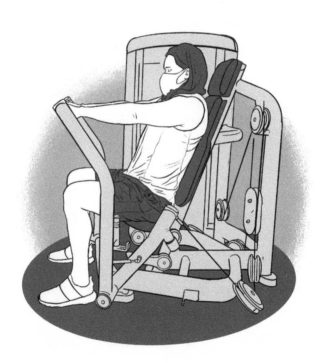

Adjustments to the Machine

There are two adjustments to make on the machine. The first is to determine how far back our elbows will go when we are at rest. There are three positions that we can choose from, using a pin. Position the pin such that that the handles are in front of your chest when you are seated. This will prevent you from hyperextending your shoulders.

The next thing to adjust is the seat's height relative to the machine. The seat height should be set so the handles line up with our chest at the same height as the lower part of the sternum. The nice thing about this machine is that the handles are not aligned perfectly straight with one another. This small angle of deflection is much more comfortable for our shoulders than a straight bar.

Stretching

Standing next to the stack of weights on the machine, we place our hand at the top of the machine with our palm facing forward, twisting our body to help stretch the pectoralis major muscle. We may have to bend our knees a little to find the right spot. Hold the stretch for twenty seconds, switch arms, and repeat.

The chest press machine puts strain on our pectoral muscles, triceps, and front shoulder muscles (deltoids). This stretch will help loosen those muscles and help our active recovery between two-minute intervals.

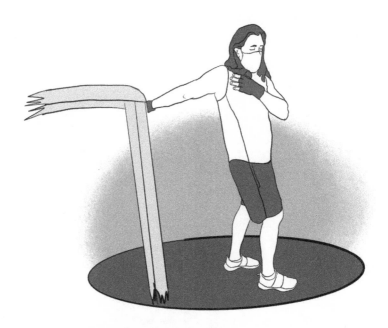

Proper Form

As we sit down, we keep our arms parallel to the motion of the handles so we are pushing with our chest. We will start with the machine at rest and our hands facing downward on the handles, gripping them like bicycle handlebars.

We visualize our chest muscles squeezing as we push out slowly. We tense up our pectoralis major when we reach the apex of the movement, then slowly bring the handles back to the starting position.

We push the whole time while letting the handles come back to the start. We want to focus on our chest muscles for the return movement rather than using our triceps, which will kick in when our chest is not the focus.

Breathing

Prior to our first movement, we let all the air out of our lungs, then take in a deep breath. As we begin slowly pushing the handles forward, we start letting the air out. Halfway through the push, we take another breath and begin letting it out slowly as we reach the apex. Another breath at the apex will give us plenty of oxygen to let the handles return slowly to the starting point. Halfway through the return motion, we take another breath.

Exercise 2: Pectoral Fly Machine

The pectoral fly machine strengthens our pectoralis major muscles. (We also use it on Day 2 to work our rear deltoids and back.)

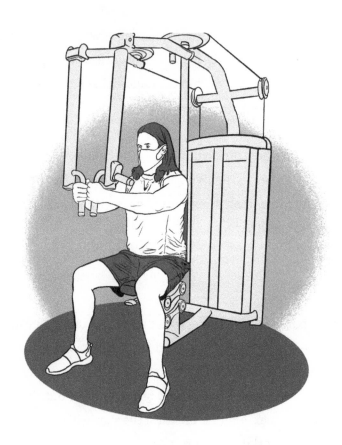

Adjustments to the Machine

The first thing to adjust is the position of the handles. We will be holding the vertical handles, and adjusting the pin at the top of the machine allows us to rotate these to keep our arms from going too far back when the machine is at rest. Adjust the pins so that when you hold the handles, your arms are straight out from your sides.

Next, adjust the seat so that the top of your hand is at or just below the height of your shoulders when your arms are parallel to the floor.

Stretching

Standing in front of the seat, grip the center pole behind the seat with your left hand at the same height as your shoulders, and turn your body to the right. Twist your body to help stretch the pectoralis major. You may have to bend your knees a little to find the right spot. Hold the stretch for twenty seconds, switch arms, and repeat.

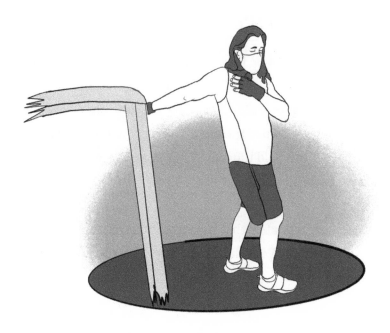

Proper Form

Sitting facing away from the machine with our hands on the handles, we push our hands forward while the machine keeps our hands moving in a circular motion as they come together in front of us. Our shoulders are the pivot point of this exercise, so we will be careful to slightly bend our arms so that we increase pressure to our pectorals, not our elbows (which are pressured when our arms are straight). We focus on our chest muscles and adjust accordingly.

Breathing

Prior to our first movement, we let all the air out of our lungs, then take in a deep breath. As we begin slowly pushing the handles forward, we start letting the air out. Halfway through the push, we take another breath, which we begin letting it out slowly as we reach the apex. Another breath at the apex will allow us to have plenty of oxygen to let the handles return slowly to the starting point. Halfway through the return motion, we take another breath.

Exercise 3: Incline Chest Press

The incline chest press machine strengthens our pectoralis minor muscles. These are the muscles at the top of our chest and are a muscle group that is often overlooked by those who do normal chest exercises. The movement is done at forty-five degrees, roughly halfway between the chest press and overhead press.

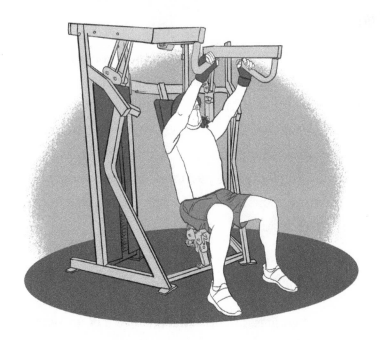

Adjustments to the Machine

The height of the seat should be such that the handles are one inch above the line crossing the lower part of our sternum. If the seat is too low, we will feel like we are putting strain on our shoulders, and if it is too high, we will feel like we are bending our wrists too much. Our wrists should be straight when we perform the movement.

Stretching

Stand behind the machine and grasp a vertical support structure just above the horizontal crossmember. With your palms facing forward, twist your body by rotating around the foot farthest from the machine so you can feel the stretch across the top of your chest. You may have to lean backward and bend your knees a bit. Hold the stretch for twenty seconds, switch arms, and repeat.

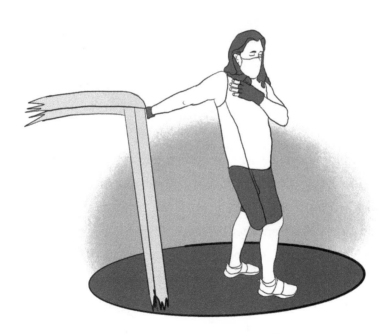

Proper Form

We sit, facing away from the machine, with our hands on the handles. We do our first set with a grip close to the ends of the handles and our hands close to the center of our chest. The second set will bring our hands farther apart to get a wider grip on the handles. The third set will have us return to the close grip. To perform the movement, we grasp the horizontal handles and, while keeping the center of our chest as the pivot point, push the handles out to fully extend our arms. We slowly return the handles to the starting position while keeping pressure on our upper chest muscles. To really stretch those, we slow down as we approach the starting position.

Breathing

Prior to our first movement, we let all the air out of our lungs and take in a deep breath. Begin slowly pushing the handles forward, and when we do, start letting the air out. Halfway through the push, we will take another breath and will begin letting it out slowly as we reach the apex. Another breath at the apex will allow us to have plenty of oxygen to let the handles return slowly to the starting point. Halfway through the return motion, we will take another breath.

Day 2: Back

Our back is made up of several distinct muscle groups. Starting at the top of our back, we have the trapezius, which is a pair of triangular muscles connecting the bottom of our skull to our shoulders and to the middle of our back. These are often referred to as our "traps"; we use them when we lift our shoulders.

Next, we have the latissimus dorsi, which connect the lower back to the lower ribs and to a tendon that connects to the top of our upper arm bone, which is called the humerus. These are the muscles that make a person look like they have a wide back. They are often referred to as the "lats," and we use them during pull-ups.

Hidden underneath our lats are a pair of muscles called the rhomboids. These connect our shoulder blades to the center of our spine. They are immensely powerful muscles that help us rotate our shoulder blades when we pull something toward us, such as a rope.

Below our lats, in what we commonly refer to as our lumbar region, is a long set of muscles called the multifidus. We will focus on the lower portion of this set of muscles, which helps with leaning forward and pulling back. Movements like rowing build this muscle group. It is important to keep this portion and the top of our gluteus muscles strong, as when they weaken, we risk "throwing our back out," which can be very painful.

The following back exercises are performed wearing lifting hooks or with bare hands, so we will only need to bring our water bottle and lifting hooks for Day 2 exercises.

Exercise 1: Back Extension

The back extension strengthens our lower back muscles, including our gluteus medius, the muscles that keep our butt higher and rounder as we age. When using this machine, we need to continue to work toward a full extension of our back. We place the center of our feet on the footrests, with our feet spaced so that we can sit straight. We keep a slight, barely perceptible bend to our knees to prevent injury. We do not use the lifting hooks on this machine.

We lean forward as we sit down, being sure to keep our head straight throughout the movement so that our back takes all the pressure. We lean back while keeping our hands on the handles with our palms facing toward our body. As we push up slowly, we visualize the muscles in our lower back pulling and squeezing our glutes. This extra bit of movement will do wonders for how our butt looks. As we slowly lean forward, coming back to the starting position, we continue to push up while letting our body come back to the start. There is a difference between letting the weight down and pushing up against it to slow it down.

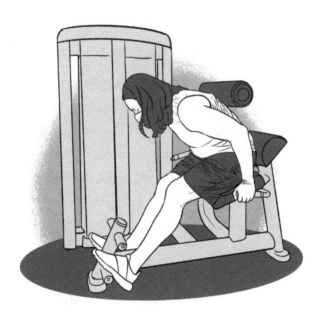

Adjustments to the Machine

An adjustable pin allows us to set the starting degree of rotation. The setting is based on how flexible we are. Over time, try to lower the starting point so you begin engaging the upper part of the lumbar spine.

Stretching

Standing with our feet about three inches apart, we place our palms together and lift them above our head while slightly leaning back. Slowly leaning forward with our legs straight, we suck in our stomach and hang, leaning down. Next, we exhale and let our back muscles stretch. Letting our hands hang will eventually allow us to touch our toes, then the floor. After a while, we can get to a place where our palms are on the ground. Do not try to stretch too far at first. It may take you many months or years to touch the floor. Stretching is not a contest. Our lower back muscles will loosen up and become more limber over time.

Hold the stretch for twenty seconds and then slowly come back upright. Take a deep breath and start again.

Proper Form

We slowly begin leaning back on the machine with our hands on the handles, palms facing inward, head straight, as it should stay throughout the movement. We lean back and slowly straighten our body until we get to the apex point. We focus on bending at the waist. We slowly lean forward until there is no remaining pressure on our back from the machine.

Breathing

Prior to our first movement, we will let all the air out of our lungs and take in a deep breath. As we begin to slowly lean backward, we will let the air out of our lungs. Halfway through the backward movement, we will take another breath and begin letting it out slowly until we reach the apex. Another breath at the apex will allow us to have plenty of oxygen to let the machine return slowly to the starting point. Halfway through the return motion, we will take another breath.

Exercise 2: Pull-Down

The pull-down machine strengthens our latissimus dorsi and teres major back muscles, the muscles that give us wings. We use the lifting hooks with this machine, so be sure to put them on before starting.

The only thing to adjust with this machine is the seat height. We adjust the seat so that we sit with our arms stretched upward and the lifting hooks hooked over the handles. Our legs will be pinned in a seated position under the padded supports.

As we sit, we pull our arms down to the sides of our body by bending them and pulling with our lats. Bringing the handles down so our hands end up just above our shoulders, we look up at the handles and slowly tilt our head forward as we pull down. Hold the handles at the bottom position for one second before slowly letting them come back up to the starting position.

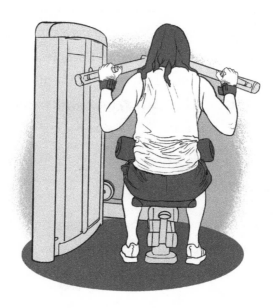

Stretching

Standing with our feet at shoulder width, we grab the center support above the seat and lean backward. Hold the stretch for twenty seconds and then slowly come back upright. Take a deep breath and start again.

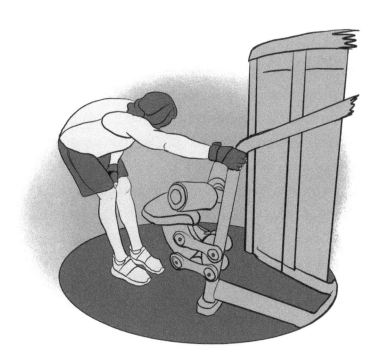

Proper Form

Being seated on the machine with our hands on the handles, palms facing forward, we keep our head straight. Slowly begin pulling the handles down until an imaginary bar connecting the handles is resting on the shoulders. Pull down and do a small crunch with your stomach muscles. Slowly let the handles come back to their starting point.

Breathing

Prior to our first movement we will let all the air out of our lungs and breathe in a deep breath. As we begin to slowly lean backward, we start letting the air out. Halfway through the backward movement, we will take another breath and begin letting it out slowly as we reach the apex. Another breath at the apex will allow us to have plenty of oxygen to let the machine return slowly to the starting point. Halfway through the return motion, we will take another breath.

Exercise 3: Rear Deltoid

The rear deltoid exercise strengthens our backward-facing shoulder muscles and the infraspinatus muscles, which sit adjacent to the deltoids. This exercise is done on the same machine as the pectoral fly. But this time, we sit facing the machine, looking at the weight stack, with arms stretched out in front, holding the handles. The machine's movement has us bring our hands to the sides of our body like Leonardo da Vinci's *Vitruvian Man*. We do not use the lifting hooks on this machine.

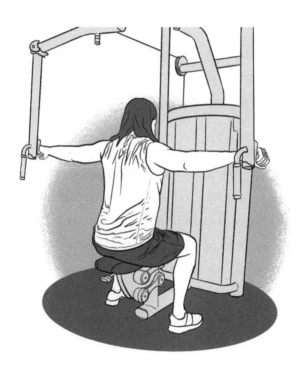

Adjustments to the Machine

Use the pins to set the starting degree of rotation and the seat position. Adjust the handles to start in the rear deltoid position by pulling the pin below the top of the handle aperture and rotating the handles to the innermost position. Letting go of the pin will allow it to snap into the right position.

The height of the seat should be set so that we can keep our arms parallel to the floor.

Stretching

Standing in front of the machine with our body facing the seat, we see a vertical tube coming up from behind the seat. With our right hand, we grip the tube just above the seat. We start to lean backward, putting all the stretch into our right arm, right shoulder, and right part of our back. Bending our legs helps us draw the stretch out. Hold the stretch for twenty seconds and then slowly come back upright. We switch to holding the tube with our left hand and repeat.

Proper Form

We start by grasping the horizontal handles with our hands facing down in front of our body. We pull our hands back so they end up outstretched to the sides. Keeping our shoulders as the pivot point, we pull our hands apart and to our sides. We slightly bend our arms so we add pressure to our back and not just our shoulder muscles. Focus on the upper back muscles and adjust accordingly.

Breathing

Prior to our first movement, we will let all the air out of our lungs and breathe in a deep breath. Slowly bringing our arms back to our sides, we start letting the air out. Halfway through the backward movement, we will take another breath and will begin letting it out slowly as we reach the apex. Another breath at the apex will allow us to have plenty of oxygen to let the machine return slowly to the starting point. Halfway through the return motion, we will take another breath.

Exercise 4: Row Machine

The row machine strengthens our upper and middle back muscles. Building strength in this area is critical because it will help us pick things up without back pain. This machine targets our upper back muscles, so we do not have to perform the leg portion of a typical row. We use the lifting hooks with this machine, so be sure to put them on before starting.

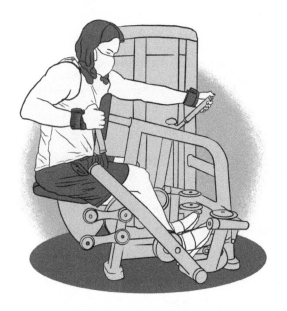

Adjustments to the Machine

The height of the seat should be such that when we hold the handles, our arms are almost completely stretched out.

We adjust the chest pad via a pin just behind it at the top of the center tube. This can be individually adjusted so when we pull back on the handles, the resistance starts right away.

Stretching

Standing facing the side of the weight stack with our feet shoulder-width apart, we grip the vertical tube on the side of the weight stack with our right hand and lean backward to stretch the upper portion of our back. We exhale as we slowly lean backward with our legs bent. Hold the stretch for twenty seconds and then slowly come back upright. Take a deep breath, switch arms, and start again.

Proper Form

Using the lifting hooks, we begin by pulling one arm back to our side, making sure not to bend our neck during this exercise. It is important to keep our back straight as we reach as far back with our elbows as is comfortable. Once we reach the apex, we hold the handles there for half a second and then slowly start returning the handles to their starting position.

Breathing

Prior to the first movement, we will let all the air out of our lungs and take in a deep breath. We begin slowly pulling the handle backward and slowly let the air out of our lungs. Halfway through the backward movement, we will take another breath and begin letting it out slowly as we reach the apex. Another breath at the apex will allow us to have plenty of oxygen to let the machine return slowly to the starting point. Halfway through the return motion, we will take another breath.

Day 3: Legs

Our leg muscles comprise several groups. We will focus on the main groupings we use in our daily life. Starting at the top of the leg in the front, we have quadriceps. On the back side of our leg at the top are the hamstrings. The sides of our shins are the tibiales, and on the back of our legs are the calves.

The following leg exercises are performed without gloves or lifting hooks, so you will only need to bring the water bottle to the gym for leg day.

Exercise 1: Leg Extension

The leg extension is used to help strengthen our quadriceps and tibialis muscles. This machine puts pressure on our knees, so it is important to warm our knees up before starting. I warm up my knees with the red light prior to going to the gym on leg day, and once I am on the machine, I cover my knees with my palms for the first set to keep my kneecaps warm, as well as the ligaments and tendons connecting them to the leg bones.

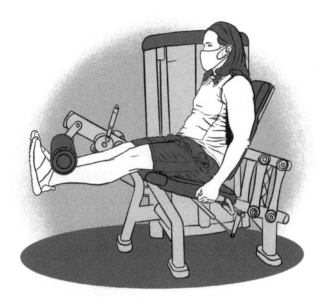

Adjustments to the Machine

The first thing to do is set the weight at five pounds so we can easily adjust the machine without risking injury. There is a pin behind the left handle whereby we can adjust the depth of the seat back. We will want to set this to something comfortable, and we will adjust it again after we do the other two adjustments.

Next, we adjust the degree of rotation so that we start with our knees bent and our feet under the seat. There is an adjustment for the height of our legs that will move a padded bar up and down. Set it so it comfortably rests at the bottom of the shin.

We now return to the pin that adjusts the seat depth and make sure that our back is well supported. Once we have this set properly, be sure to set the proper weight for today's lift.

Stretching

Standing on our left foot, with our right hand gripping the seat, we bend our left leg and reach back to grab our shin or foot. We slowly pull the foot back so that it stretches the quadriceps. Hold the stretch for twenty seconds and then slowly come back upright. Take a deep breath, and start again with the other leg.

Proper Form

Seated on the machine with our hands gripping the handles, our palms facing inward, and our back and head straight, we slowly begin straightening our legs. Once they are completely straight, we hold it for a half second and then slowly begin bending them back to the starting position. There are two versions of the movement. We can keep our feet at ninety-degree angles, or we can point our toes as we bring up the weight. I like to switch between the two for each repetition so I can work different supporting muscles.

Breathing

Prior to our first movement, we will let all the air out of our lungs and take in a deep breath. We start slowly letting out the air as we begin slowly straightening our legs. Another breath at the apex will allow us to have plenty of oxygen to let the machine return slowly to the starting point. Halfway through the return motion, we may want to take another breath, depending on the speed of our movement.

Exercise 2: Seated Leg Curl

The seated leg curl strengthens our hamstrings. This machine is the opposite movement of the leg extension machine and should be done right after the leg extension, to balance the muscle strain on our legs.

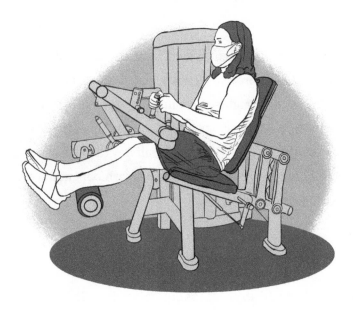

Adjustments to the Machine

This one takes a little practice setting up. The first thing to do is set the weight at five pounds so we can adjust the machine to our body. There is a pin behind the seat whereby we can adjust the depth of the seat. We initially set this to something comfortable, and we will adjust it again after we have set three other adjustments.

Next, we adjust the degree of rotation so we are starting with our legs straight but not hyperextended. It is okay to have a small bend in our knees when we are seated. There is an adjustment for the height of our legs that will move the padded bar up and down. Set it so that it comfortably rests at our Achilles tendon, just above our shoes.

After the leg height is adjusted, we adjust the pin to lower the top bar so that it rests on the top of our legs. You may feel a little pressure from the bar. Once we have that set, we go back to the pin that adjusts the seat depth to make sure our back is well supported. Once we have it set properly, be sure to set the proper weight for today's lift.

Stretching

Standing with our feet about three inches apart, we place our palms together and lift them above our head while slightly leaning back. We suck in our stomach as we slowly lean forward with our legs straight. We exhale and let our back muscles stretch as our hands hang. We will be able to touch our toes or the floor, and with practice our palms can rest on the ground. Do not try to stretch too far at first. It may take many months or years to touch the floor. There is no contest in stretching. It is all about getting in a proper stretch. Over time, we will loosen up our lower back muscles and will become much more limber.

Hold the stretch for twenty seconds and slowly come back upright. Take a deep breath and start again.

Proper Form

We sit on the machine, gripping the handles on the bar above our legs, palms facing inward. Keeping our back and head straight and our legs straight out in front, we slowly begin curling our legs under the seat by pushing against the bar. Focusing on curling as far as we can, we hold the position for a half second and then slowly start releasing the curl. There are two versions of the movement. We can either keep our feet at ninety-degree angles or we can point our toes as we bend our legs. I like to switch between the two for each repetition so I can work different supporting muscles.

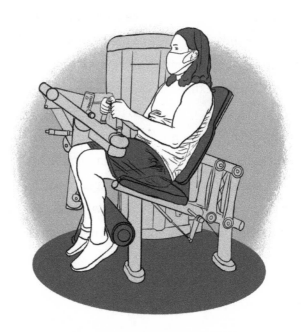

Breathing

Prior to our first movement, we will let all the air out of our lungs and take in a deep breath. We slowly let the air out of our lungs as we begin slowly curling our legs. Another breath at the apex will allow us to have plenty of oxygen to let the machine return slowly to the starting point. Halfway through the return motion, we may want to take another breath, depending on the speed of our movement.

Exercise 3: Calf Extension

The calf extension is used to help strengthen our calf muscles and the muscles in our feet. The key to making this machine work well for us is to get the seat set to the proper depth so we have a small bend to our knees when the machine is at rest.

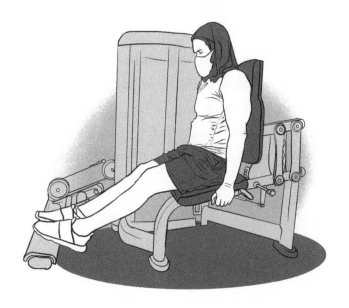

Adjustments to the Machine

There is a pin behind the left handle of the machine whereby we can adjust the depth of the seat back. We will want to set this so that when we have our feet on the foot pad, our knees are slightly bent.

Stretching

Standing behind the seat near the weight rack, we place the ball of our right foot against the lower crossmember, with the heel of our shoe touching the floor. Then we will lean forward, with our left foot behind us. Keeping our right leg straight as we lean, the calf of our right leg will stretch. We hold the stretch for twenty seconds and then slowly reduce the angle of our lean. Take a deep breath and start again with the other leg.

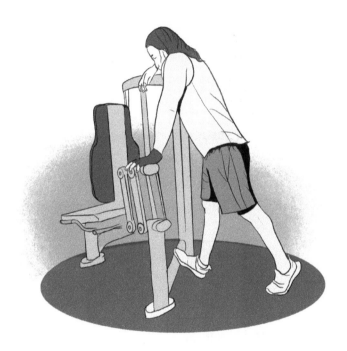

Proper Form

We sit on the machine with our hands gripping the handles, palms facing inward, and our back and head straight. Next, we place our feet six inches apart on the foot pad and slowly begin pushing the footrest by pointing our toes, straightening our legs completely, with our toes pointing forward, until we reach the apex. Hold at the apex for a half second and then slowly start releasing the pressure against the foot pad. There are three versions of the movement. We can keep our feet parallel as we push, point our toes inward at a fifteen-degree angle, or point our toes outward at a fifteen-degree angle. I prefer to do one set of each.

Breathing

Prior to the first movement, we let all the air out of our lungs and take in a deep breath. We begin slowly pointing our toes when we do start letting the air out. Another breath at the apex will allow us to have plenty of oxygen to let the machine return slowly to the starting point. Halfway through the return motion, we may want to take another breath, depending on the speed of our movement.

Exercise 4: Seated Leg Press

The seated leg press strengthens our quadriceps, glutes, and hamstrings. This machine puts pressure on our knees, so it is important to warm them up before starting. I like to use the red light on my knees before going to the gym. Once at the gym, we can place our palms on our kneecaps and ligaments to keep them warm as we start.

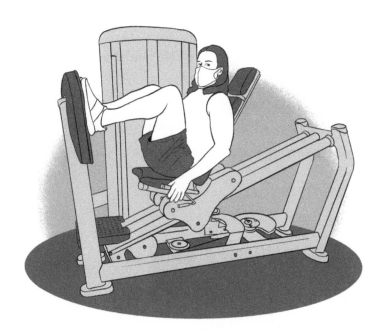

Adjustments to the Machine

First we set the weight at five pounds, as always. There is a handle that will disengage a ratchet-and-pawl mechanism that sets the seat height. To set it correctly, we pull the handle and set the height so that our legs are at a ninety-degree angle when we feel pressure on the movement.

Stretching

Standing on our left foot, with our left hand gripping the seat, we bend our left leg and reach back to grab our shin or foot. Slowly and gently pull the foot back so that it stretches our quadriceps. Hold for twenty seconds and then slowly come back upright. Take a deep breath and start again with the other leg.

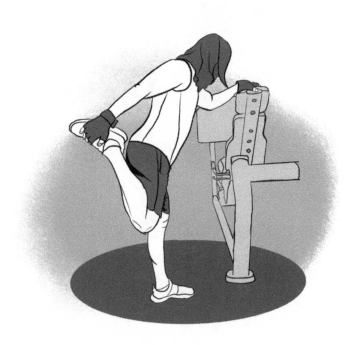

Proper Form

We sit on the machine with our hands gripping the handles, palms facing inward, and our back and head straight. We set our feet at shoulder width on the large foot pad, with our toes pointed slightly outward. We slowly begin straightening our legs until they are completely straight, hold for a half second and then slowly start bending them back to the starting position.

Breathing

Prior to the first movement, we let all the air out of our lungs and take in a deep breath. We begin slowly straightening our legs, and when we do, start letting the air out. Another breath at the apex will allow us to have plenty of oxygen to let the machine return slowly to the starting point. Halfway through the return motion, we may want to take another breath, depending on the speed of our movement.

Day 4: Arms

Our arm muscles comprise several groups. Starting at the top and in the front, we have the biceps. *Bicep* is from the Latin for "two heads." The full name is musculus biceps brachii or "two-headed muscle of the arm." There are indeed two heads on the muscle group, the long head and the short head. The long head is what gives weightlifters that big ball of muscle when they flex. We can change which head we work by adjusting our grip. A wide grip when performing curls works the short head; a narrow grip, the long head.

At the top of the back of the arm is the triceps. This is from the Latin for "three-headed muscle of the arm." These are made up of the long, medial, and lateral heads. We will work each.

Below our elbow is the forearm. There are six muscles that overlay or are adjacent to each other. These allow our hand to move up and down.

Do the following arm exercises, if possible, in the following order. And wear gloves for all of them.

Exercise 1: Seated Biceps Curl Machine

The seated biceps curl machine strengthens our biceps and forearm muscles by enabling us to do curls without using dumbbells.

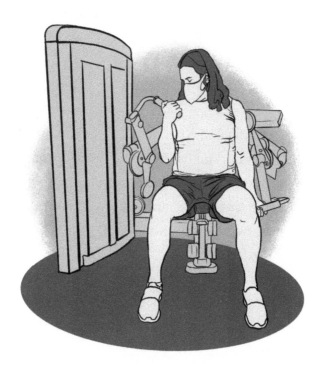

Adjustments to the Machine

The first thing to do is set the weight at five pounds. Then we adjust the seat so we can comfortably hold the handles and move the weight through the full range of motion.

Stretching

Sitting on the machine with our arms out straight, we weave our fingers together and then turn our hands with the palms facing outward, squeezing our elbows together to stretch the biceps. Hold for twenty seconds and then slowly release. Take a deep breath and start again.

Proper Form

Seated on the machine with our right hand gripping the handle, palm facing upward, and our back and head straight, slowly begin curling the right arm. We curl our arm completely, holding it for a half second at the apex, and then slowly start stretching out our arm. Do two minutes on each arm.

There are two versions of the movement. We can either grip the handles close to our body to work the short head of the biceps or away from our body to work the long head. Vary the grip for each set to work both heads.

Breathing

Prior to the first movement, we let all the air out of our lungs and take in a deep breath. We begin slowly curling our arm, and when we do, start letting the air out. Another breath at the apex will allow us to have plenty of oxygen to let the machine return slowly to the starting point. Halfway through the return motion, we may want to take another breath, depending on the speed of our movement.

Exercise 2: Rope Pull-Down

The rope pull-down strengthens our triceps and forearms. This machine puts pressure on our elbows and shoulders, so it is important to warm these up before starting. I warm up by making circular motions with my arms and then bending and straightening them. Using the red light on our elbows and shoulders before going to the gym can help warm them up too.

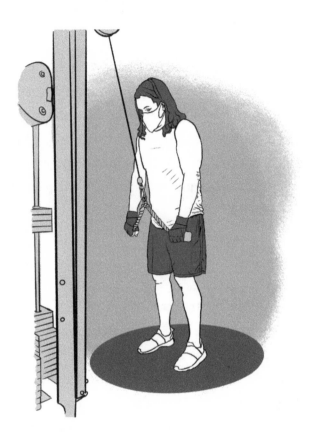

Adjustments to the Machine

Before we start, we adjust the height of the pulley where the rope attaches. The first thing to do is set the weight at five pounds. Behind the pulley, there is a pin with which we can adjust the height of the rope. You will want to set the height so your arms are bent slightly past ninety degrees when grabbing the rope.

Stretching

We stand and slowly curl our right arm while making a fist, being sure to bend our wrist inward. We slowly straighten our arm and rotate the wrist so our hand is now facing away from us with the back of the hand pointed upward. We try to extend our elbow while squeezing the triceps. It takes practice, but once you get it, it will be easy. Hold the stretch for twenty seconds and then slowly relax the arm. Take a deep breath and do the other arm.

Proper Form

We stand in front of the machine with our feet shoulder-width apart and our back straight. Bending slightly at the waist, we grasp each handle, with our pinky fingers resting against the rubber ball at the bottom of the rope. Starting with our hands together, as we pull the rope down, we slowly begin pulling our hands apart. We feel the pressure on our triceps. As we reach the apex, we pull our hands apart so they are farthest apart at the apex. The rope will be slightly straightened, and depending on how far apart we have our hands, the top of our triceps will feel the squeeze. The farther apart, the more squeeze you will feel. We will hold that squeeze for a half second, then slowly start bringing our hands back to the starting position. There are two versions of the movement. We can keep our hands on the rope, or we can make a modified "okay" sign with our fingers, using only our thumb, pointer finger, and middle finger to hold the rope. I like to switch from set to set to work different supporting muscles.

Exercise 3: Biceps Curl

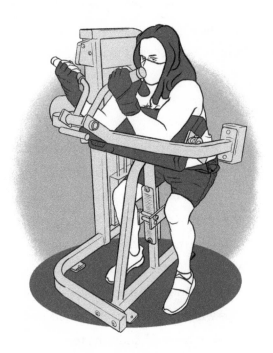

The biceps curl machine strengthens our biceps and forearm muscles. It simulates the seated barbell curl without putting too much pressure on our back and elbows.

Adjustments to the Machine

The seat is held at an angle, and when we pull the seat up, it will click into place. Pull up and out on the seat to lower it. The first thing to do is set the weight at five pounds. We adjust the seat so our armpits rest against the large pad and our arms can comfortably reach the handles and make the full rotational movement.

Stretching

Sitting on the machine with our arms out straight, we weave our fingers together and then turn our hands with the palms facing outward, squeezing our elbows together to stretch the biceps. Hold for twenty seconds and then slowly release. Take a deep breath and start again.

Proper Form

Seated on the machine with our hands gripping the handles, palms facing upward, and our back and head straight, we slowly begin curling our arms to bring the handle toward our head. Once we curl our arms completely, we hold it for a half second and then slowly start lowering our arms, making sure to keep pressure on the handles until they come back to the starting position.

Breathing

Prior to the first movement, we let all the air out of our lungs and take in a deep breath. We begin slowly curling our arms, and when we do, we start letting the air out. Another breath at the apex will allow us to have plenty of oxygen to let the machine return slowly to the starting point. Halfway through the return motion, we may want to take another breath, depending on the speed of our movement.

Exercise 4: Triceps Press Machine

The triceps press machine strengthens our triceps and chest muscles. We push down and straighten our arms to simulate a parallel bar press. This is one of my favorite exercises because it strengthens my shoulders and triceps like no other.

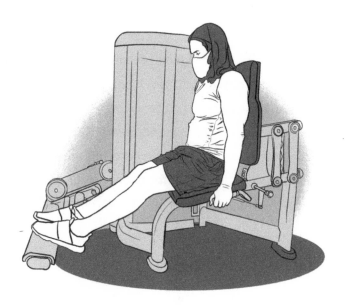

Adjustments to the Machine

The first thing to do is set the weight at five pounds. We adjust the seat so we can comfortably hold on to the handles and move the weight through the full range of motion.

Next, we rotate the handles outward to put them in their widest position. We will rotate them inward for the second set and outward again for the third set.

Stretching

We stand, make a fist, and slowly curl our right arm, making sure to bend our wrist inward. We slowly straighten our arm and rotate the wrist so our hand faces away from us with the back facing upward. We try to extend our elbow with a focus on squeezing the triceps. It takes practice, but once you get it, it will be easy. Hold the stretch for twenty seconds and then slowly relax the arm. Take a deep breath and do the other arm.

Proper Form

Sitting with our feet shoulder-width apart and our back straight, we lean our head slightly forward. Our palms facing downward, we grasp the handles from above and slowly push them until our arms are fully extended. When we reach the apex, we hold for a half second and then slowly bring the handles back to the starting position. We can also hold the handles so that our wrists are straight and our palms are facing inward.

There are two versions of the movement. We can either keep the handles outward or rotate them so they flip upside down for the inward position. I like alternating from set to set, starting with the wide position.

Breathing

Prior to the first movement, we will let all the air out of our lungs and take in a deep breath. We begin slowly pushing the handles down, and as we do, start letting the air out. Another breath at the bottom position of the handles will allow us to have plenty of oxygen to let the machine return slowly to the starting point. Halfway through the return motion, we may want to take another breath, depending on the speed of our movement.

Day 5: Shoulders

Although they have been worked out on previous days, we focus a full day on our shoulders, which comprise a group of muscles called the deltoids. The deltoid is a triangular muscle that gets its name from its shape like the Greek letter delta. Our shoulders are important on their own, but they are also a key muscle group for our chest, back, and arms. Dedicating a full day to our shoulders ensures that our entire system builds strength at once.

As on every other day, remember to select at least one abdominal exercise to go with the shoulder workout to maintain consistency and strength. The exercises we will complete for our shoulders require gloves and lifting hooks. Be sure to bring them, along with your water bottle.

Exercise 1: Shoulder Press

The shoulder press strengthens the front part of our shoulders, with a bit of work on our upper chest muscles. It simulates the barbell shoulder press, also known as a "military press." We will not be able to increase our weight as easily on shoulder workouts because our shoulders have already been pivotal in our chest and arm workouts.

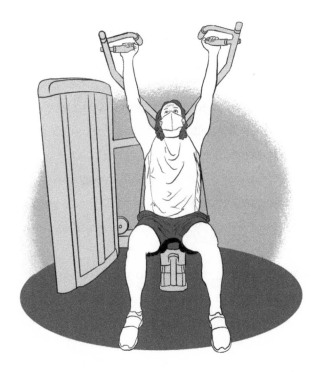

Adjustments to the Machine

We want the handles about one inch above our shoulders so that when we grab them, an imaginary bar rests on our traps.

Stretching

Standing next to the stack of weights on the machine, we place our hands at the top of the machine with our palms facing forward. We twist our body to help stretch the pectoralis major muscle and then rotate our shoulders, so we feel the stretch in our shoulders. We may have to bend our knees a little to find the right spot. We should feel the stretch in the front portion of our shoulders. Hold for twenty seconds, switch arms, and repeat.

Proper Form

As we sit down, we keep our hands on the handles and our back and head straight. We begin slowly pushing the handles up until we reach the apex. As we move the handles up, we slowly start looking up at the apex.

The key is to visualize our shoulder muscles squeezing as we push up slowly. Once we reach the apex of the movement, we hold for a half second and then slowly bring the handles back to the starting position.

We push the whole time we are letting the handles come back to the start. By focusing on our shoulder muscles during the return movement, we can keep the resistance on our shoulders rather than our triceps, which will kick in when our shoulders are not the focus.

Breathing

Prior to the first movement, we will let all the air out of our lungs and take in a deep breath. We begin slowly pushing the handles upward and start letting the air out. Halfway through the push, we will take another breath and will begin letting it out slowly as we reach the apex. Another breath at the apex will allow us to have plenty of oxygen to let the handles return slowly to the starting point. Halfway through the return motion, we will take another breath.

Exercise 2: Lateral Raise

The lateral raise strengthens the main part of our shoulder muscles. The seated position keeps us comfortable, while the split handles eliminate any chance of pressure on other muscles.

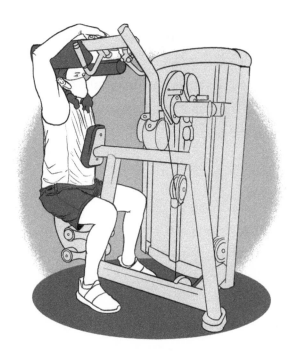

Adjustments to the Machine

We start by pulling the handle to adjust the seat height so the pads rest against our arms, just above our elbows, and the pivot point is comfortably set at the level of our shoulders.

Stretching

Standing next to the stack of weights, we place our right hand at the top of the machine with our palm facing forward. We twist our body counterclockwise to stretch the pectoral major muscle and then rotate our shoulder so that it focuses the stretch on our shoulder. We then rotate our hand so the back of it presses against the vertical support. We may have to bend our knees a little to find the right spot. Hold the stretch for twenty seconds, switch arms, and repeat.

Proper Form

As we sit down, we keep our arms on the handles and our back and head straight, and begin slowly pushing the handles out and up until we reach the apex.

We visualize our shoulder muscles squeezing as we push up slowly. Once we reach the apex, we hold for a half second and then slowly bring the handles back to the starting position.

We push the whole time we are letting the padded bars come back to the start. We focus on our shoulder muscles during the return movement rather than just letting the weight collapse.

For the second set, we sit backward on the machine. The movement will not go as high as the one we did in the forward-facing position. In this position, we work the part of our shoulders just above our triceps.

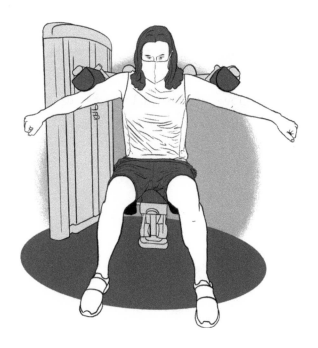

Breathing

Prior to the first movement, we let all the air out of our lungs and take in a deep breath. We begin slowly pushing the handles upward, and when we do, we start letting the air out. Another breath at the apex will allow us to have plenty of oxygen to let the handles return slowly to the starting point. Halfway through the return motion, we may have to take another breath.

Exercise 3: Cable Row Shrug

The cable row shrug strengthens our trapezius muscles. It simulates the barbell shoulder shrug. We wear lifting hooks for this exercise, so no gloves are needed. Be sure to use a straight bar so your hands can be at shoulder width and the hooks can grip without slipping.

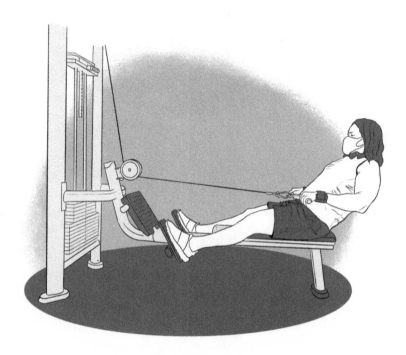

Adjustments to the Machine

There are no adjustments to this machine.

Stretching

We start standing up with our arms at our sides. Keeping our hands at our sides, we raise our shoulders and rotate them back and down in a circular motion. Once we get to the bottom, we reverse the direction and rotate up and forward. Rotate them backward and then forward in five big sweeping movements.

Proper Form

We sit on the large pad with our palms and lifting hooks facing downward. Then we straighten our legs and pull our hands to our waist as we lift our shoulders up into a shrug. We begin rotating our shoulders in a circular motion, as we did when stretching before this exercise. We perform five shrug circles before bringing the bar to the starting point and bending our legs to remove any pressure on our body.

There are three versions of this exercise. We can bring our shoulders straight up, rotate them in forward circles, or rotate them in backward circles. I recommend one set of each.

Breathing

Prior to our first movement, we let all the air out of our lungs and then take in a deep breath. We begin to slowly pull the bar, and when we do, we start letting the air out. Another breath at the apex of each circular motion will allow us to have plenty of oxygen to finish the movement. Keep breathing through the return motion.

Exercise 4: Inner Shoulder Press

The inner shoulder press strengthens the front part of our shoulders and uses the same machine as the regular shoulder press. The only difference is that we will be using the inner handles.

Adjustments to the Machine

Adjust the seat height so that the handles are about one inch above our shoulders and when we grab them, it is like we are holding two bars on our shoulders.

Stretching

Standing next to the stack of weights, we place our right hand at the top of the machine with our palm facing forward. We twist our body counterclockwise to stretch the pectoralis major and then rotate our shoulder to feel the stretch there. We may have to bend our knees a little to find the right spot. We should feel the stretch in the front of our shoulder. Hold for twenty seconds, switch arms, and repeat.

Proper Form

As we sit, we keep our hands on the inner handles and our back and head straight. As we begin slowly pushing the handles up, we look upward until we reach the apex.

We visualize our shoulder muscles squeezing as we push up slowly. Once we reach the apex, we hold for a half second and then slowly bring the handles back to the starting position.

Breathing

Prior to the first movement, we will let all the air out of our lungs and take in a deep breath. We will begin slowly pushing the handles upward, and when we do, start letting the air out. Halfway through the push, we will take another breath and will begin letting it out slowly as we reach the apex. Another breath at the apex will allow us to have plenty of oxygen to let the handles return slowly to the starting point. Halfway through the return motion, we will take another breath.

Abdominals Every Day

It is important to work our abdominal muscles each day we are at the gym. A strong core is essential for a strong body and will reduce injuries. The abdominal muscles complement the back muscles, so the easiest way to get a strong back is to work the abdominals.

Moreover, working the abdominals will help ensure mobility and prevent injury in your daily life. Without a strong core, you are more likely to lose your balance and sustain life-changing falls. As we age, one fall can make all the difference, so it is important that we never skip core exercises.

Unlike the rest of the workout, we will not perform abdominal exercises slowly. We will still perform them over the two minutes, but at a pace of about one full movement every five to six seconds. You will find your pace over your first few sets.

You will find a variety of abdominal exercises at the gym. I will give one example, but try different machines to see which work best for you. The torso rotation machine works the sides of our abs and can make a great addition to your workout.

Exercise Option: Abdominal Machine

The abdominal machine works our center abdominal muscles to strengthen the rectus abdominis muscles, which make up the "six-pack."

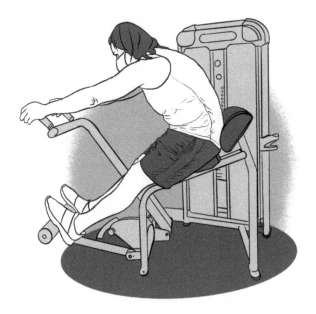

Adjustments to the Machine

We set the footrest so our back rests against the pad above the seat. This ensures we are bending at the waist. Setting the machine to five pounds, we adjust the footrest for our leg height.

Stretching

Standing with our hands above our head, we start to slowly lean backward, feeling our stomach muscles stretch. We may have to bend our knees a little to find the right spot. Hold for twenty seconds and repeat.

Proper Form

We center our feet on the footrest and sit straight. As we sit, we grip the handles, with our palms facing inward and our back and head straight. Once we begin, we straighten our arms and push against the bars by bending at the waist. Keeping our back, head, and arms straight, we sit up by pushing the handles forward. Our shoulders rotate as we move forward while keeping our arms straight. We keep a small, barely perceptible bend in our knees to prevent our legs from locking.

Breathing

We take a breath in when we are leaning backward and slowly push the air out as we lean forward. We start taking in another breath when we are fully extended, so our lungs will be full when we return to the starting point and are ready to start breathing out again.

MEDITATION FOR PET SCANS

PET scans are quite scary. Doctors use a thick, lead-lined syringe to inject radioactive sugars into our bloodstream. We must drink an entire sports drink within a few minutes, after which we wait for an hour in a small room by our-selves, without any device or other person to distract us or calm our nerves. I learned very quickly that this waiting period creates a lot of nervous energy, which I wanted, and needed, to avoid. To help myself calm down, I created a meditation routine that I hope can also help you if you are ever in the same position.

First, have the nurse turn the lights down as low as pos-sible; bright fluorescent lights can add to our stress.

We start by closing our eyes and inhaling slowly and deeply through our nose. Picture the air clean and fresh, free of any particulates. We let the air sit in our lungs a few seconds, then blow it out very slowly, keeping our eyes closed. Listen to the noise the air makes as it leaves the body.

With our eyes still closed, we picture small gray specks of dust leaving our mouth as we exhale. These gray bits are any traces of cancer still left in our body. As we exhale, they fall to the floor. We keep inhaling through our nose and exhaling through our mouth for the remainder of the hour.

We slow our breathing to relax as much as possible over the hour. It is important to keep our eyes closed through this so that our brain can focus on visualizing what we want to happen rather than processing what our eyes see in the room.

When the nurse comes to get you, simply stand up and walk into the exam room. Leave all that dust on the floor as you exit. You've got this. You are going to do great.

A NOTE ON MUSCLE FAILURE

Let us talk about muscle failure in more detail. It is critical to visualize what it means for your body. During a muscle failure, our muscle fibers and small blood vessels tear, filling the injured area with fresh blood. Our body creates inflammatory cells, which come to our muscles via the bloodstream. Muscle tissue begins to seal off the area, making sure the destruction and subsequent repair phases only occur within the affected muscles. This process starts within the first few days after each workout. That is why we only work each primary muscle group once a week.

The process of sealing off muscles starts the repair phase, necessary for muscle growth, in which a worker cell known as a macrophage finds its way to the affected muscle and cleans away any dead tissue like a vacuum cleaner.

After the dead tissue is removed from the area, cells of another type are released into the bloodstream, and once they reach the muscle, they convert themselves into myoblast cells. These group together with cells called fibroblasts, creating new muscle fibers and connective tissue. This is why our muscles grow over time when we are training with weights.

The repair process creates new blood vessels, which bring more blood to the muscle. The increase in blood and blood flow means improved muscular efficiency of adenosine triphosphate (ATP) production in the mitochondria. ATP is the source of energy that powers muscle contractions. The increase in blood flow also helps remove waste products such as ammonia and other metabolites, allowing our body to recover more quickly. This is one reason we drink so much water in the FitFAB Workout—doing so increases our blood's ability to move these blood cells around.

While our muscles repair themselves, they also change their shape through a process called muscle remodeling. New muscle fibers continue to mature and orient themselves within the muscle during this phase. These new tissues tend to be out of alignment with existing muscle fibers. Therefore, we tend to feel sore as our muscles grow, which is why stretching is so important to aligning our new muscle tissue. We do a lot of stretching during our workouts to prevent soreness and future injuries.

CONCLUSION

The FitFAB Workout saved my life, three times. It has allowed me to thrive in the most stressful situations by giving me a framework for calming my mind and strengthening my body. By no longer flying by the seat of my pants with no structure at the gym, I have been able to focus on clearing the negativity that results from a health crisis.

The FitFAB story is about you, seen through my eyes and via my words. I am your Sherpa, guiding you up the mountain that is the modern-day gym.

The goal of this book is to provide a framework that allows you to comfortably enter the gym each day with a game plan. Though stringent in its fundamentals, the framework is flexible in its implementation. Each person's body is different, and some people have previous injuries that prevent them from performing certain movements. This is where I encourage you to innovate within the framework.

For example, consider the ratio of initial movement duration to return movement duration. This can be adjusted, and I have tried a lot of variations. You may prefer a ratio of one to one, or you may favor a high-low variation, which is five seconds out and fifteen seconds on the return, or the low-high variation, which is fifteen seconds out and five seconds on the return. Each variation can benefit your muscles, depending on your overall goal.

Another way to innovate is to switch exercises for a given body part. I enjoy incorporating hip abduction and adduction machines to work my inner and outer leg muscles, so I add those machines occasionally, and when I do, I stay at the gym twenty minutes longer. There are also various abdominal machines you can add in place of the abdominal machine I discuss in this book.

There are two aspects of the regimen that I strongly discourage you from varying. The first is the rest period at the end of the return movement. You may be tempted to not let your muscles rest and go right back into the new repetition. This puts a lot of pressure on your muscles and your powerband will decrease drastically, which can lead to permanent joint injuries.

The second is the type of exercise I describe in this book. We use machines that protect you in case of muscle failure, fatigue, or injury. You can get extraordinarily strong using this framework, but if you begin using free weights with it, a dropped bar on your clavicle may permanently hurt you. Stick with machines that use cables, levers, pivot points, or stacked weights, as these have no chance of falling on you or your feet.

Please dedicate yourself to maintaining the muscle strength and peace of mind that are the main benefits of the FitFAB Workout.

Are you willing to start your FitFAB journey? There is no better time than now. You cannot injure yourself when you start out with just five pounds. I ask of you nothing I have not done myself. Start today by ordering the equipment listed in the book and getting your gym membership ready. We are going to do this. I am in this with you.

You can find more information on which items to order, applications that may make your gym life easier, and the *Fit for Any Battle* podcast at my website, fitforanybattle.com.

I would love to see pictures of you as you progress through your FitFAB journey. Please consider tagging me on Twitter (@ fitforanybattle). I wish you great success in your journey, and if you ever want to reach out to me, please visit my website for contact information.

Have I told you that I am proud of you? Well, I am.

Now ready, steady, lift!

Richard Bagdonas

ACKNOWLEDGMENTS

Writing this book was cathartic, as it helped me focus on fitness as I went through cancer treatment and recovery from COVID-19. While countless people have supported me along the way, I would like to take a moment to recognize a few who were instrumental in getting this book into your hands.

I would not have been able to write this book without the emotional and artistic support of my beautiful and talented wife, Tina Schweiger. She hand-drew each illustration in this book while simultaneously running a company and studying for her master's degree at Harvard. She was incredibly supportive of my mission to build and test the FitFAB Workout from our home in East Austin. Thank you, sweetness!

I would like to thank my friend Jordan Thaeler for being one of the guinea pigs for the workout and a second set of eyes on the original content.

I would like to thank Willie Benoit and the members of the CapTex Cruisers for helping me keep my cardio up each Thursday as we pedal around Austin.

I would like to thank the staff members of Planet Fitness in Austin for their gracious hospitality as we tested the FitFAB Workout in their facility over the last five years.

ABOUT THE AUTHOR

RICHARD BAGDONAS is a weightlifter, a bodybuilder, the creator of the FitFAB mobile app, and your personal fitness sherpa leading you through the FitFAB program.

Richard has a passion for creating systems. His greatest accomplishment is Operation Turkey—procuring and moving food to those who need it most on Thanksgiving. Richard and tens of thousands of volunteers now feed more than 15 percent of America's homeless and less fortunate populations.

Born in New York and raised in Southern California, he has been living in Austin, Texas, since the mid '90s. Today, Richard lives in East Austin with his amazing wife, Tina, and their two handsome sons and two adorable dogs.

To learn more about FitFAB and connect with Richard visit fitforanybattle.com.

CPSIA information can be obtained
at www.ICGtesting.com
Printed in the USA
LVHW090615160122
708633LV00004B/13/J